D0290312

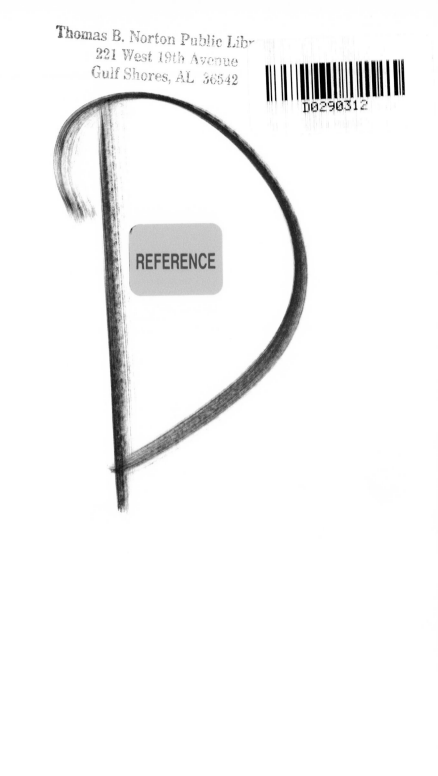

REFERENCE

Healthy Heart
SOURCEBOOK
for Women

Health Reference Series

First Edition

Healthy Heart
SOURCEBOOK
for Women

*Basic Consumer Health Information
about Cardiac Issues Specific to Women,
Including Facts about Major Risk Factors and
Prevention, Treatment and Control Strategies,
and Important Dietary Issues:*

*Along with a Special Section Regarding the
Pros and Cons of Hormone Replacement
Therapy and Its Impact on Heart Health,
and Additional Help, Including Recipes,
a Glossary, and a Directory of Resources*

Edited by
Dawn D. Matthews

Omnigraphics

615 Griswold Street • Detroit, MI 48226

Bibliographic Note

Because this page cannot legibly accommodate all the copyright notices, the Bibliographic Note portion of the Preface constitutes an extension of the copyright notice.

Beginning with books published in 1999, each new volume of the *Health Reference Series* has been individually titled and called a "First Edition." Subsequent updates will carry sequential edition numbers. To help avoid confusion and to provide maximum flexibility in our ability to respond to informational needs, the practice of consecutively numbering each volume has been discontinued.

Edited by Dawn D. Matthews

Health Reference Series

Karen Bellenir, *Series Editor*
Peter D. Dresser, *Managing Editor*
Joan Margeson, *Research Associate*
Dawn Matthews, *Verification Assistant*
Margaret Mary Missar, *Research Coordinator*
Jenifer Swanson, *Research Associate*

EdIndex, *Indexers*

Omnigraphics, Inc.

Matthew P. Barbour, *Vice President, Operations*
Laurie Lanzen Harris, *Vice President, Editorial Director*
Kevin Hayes, *Production Coordinator*
Thomas J. Murphy, *Vice President, Finance and Comptroller*
Peter E. Ruffner, *Senior Vice President*
Jane J. Steele, *Marketing Consultant*

Frederick G. Ruffner, Jr., Publisher

© 2000, Omnigraphics, Inc.

Library of Congress Cataloging-in-Publication Data

Library of Congress Cataloging-in-Publication Data

The healthy heart sourcebook for women : basic consumer health information about cardiac issues specific to women ... / edited by Dawn D. Matthews.-- 1st ed.
  p. cm. -- (Health reference series)
Includes bibliographical references and index.
ISBN 0-7808-0329-9 (lib. bdg. : acid-free paper)
  1. Heart disease in women--Popular works. I. Matthews, Dawn D. II. Series.

RC672 .H386 2000
616.1'2'0082--dc21

00-021143

∞

This book is printed on acid-free paper meeting the ANSI Z39.48 Standard. The infinity symbol that appears above indicates that the paper in this book meets that standard.

Table of Contents

Part III: Treatment and Control Strategies

Part IV: The Hormone Replacement Therapy Controversy

Part V: Dietary Issues and Cardiac Health

Part VI: Additional Help and Information

Preface

About This Book

Each year, about 370,000 women die of heart disease, making it the number one killer of American women. Some risk factors, such as age and heredity, cannot be controlled; but many others, including high blood cholesterol, high blood pressure, obesity, a sedentary lifestyle, and smoking, can be managed to help women maintain health.

Healthy Heart Sourcebook for Women tells readers why they should be concerned about heart health and what to do to prevent heart disease. It discusses the controversy surrounding hormone replacement therapy (HRT) as it relates to heart disease and breast cancer. It includes a section on dietary issues and cardiac health along with some sample "heart healthy" recipes. A glossary of important terms and a resource section provide additional help and information.

How to Use This Book

This book is divided into parts and chapters. Parts focus on broad areas of interest. Chapters are devoted to single topics within a part.

Part I: Introduction to Women and Heart Disease offers statistics about the incidence of heart disease in women, a personal quiz to help determine individual risk factors, and a chapter on heart anatomy.

Part II: Major Risk Factors and Prevention takes a more in-depth look at the risks of heart disease to women and discusses important prevention issues.

Part III: Treatment and Control Strategies offers information about women and heart attacks and the treatment strategies involved.

Part IV: The Hormone Replacement Therapy Controversy discusses the pros and cons of hormone replacement therapy (HRT). It also offers an informative chapter on synthetic hormones.

Part V: Dietary Issues and Cardiac Health contains information about nutrition as it relates to cardiac health. Some sample recipes are provided.

Part VI: Additional Help and Information includes a glossary of important terms and resources for further help and information.

Bibliographic Note

This volume contains documents and excerpts from publications issued by the following government agencies: National Heart, Lung, and Blood Institute (NHLBI); National Institute of Mental Health (NIHM), National Institutes of Health (NIH); United States Department of Agriculture (USDA); United States Department of Health and Human Services (DHHS); United States Food and Drug Administration (FDA); and the Weight Control Information Network (WCIN).

In addition, this volume contains copyrighted articles from The American Medical Association (AMA); Center for Medical Consumers, Inc.; Environmental Nutrition, Inc.; John Hopkins University; John Wiley & Sons; Harvard Medical School Health; Hippocrates, Inc.; Kettering Medical Center; Lancet, Ltd.; Lyda Associates, Inc.; MacLean Hunter Ltd., (Canada); Medical Economics Publishing; Norton Hospital; Springhouse Corp.; and Tufts University.

Full citation information is provided on the first page of each chapter. Every effort has been made to secure all necessary rights to reprint the copyrighted material. If any omissions have been made, please contact Omnigraphics to make corrections for future editions.

Acknowledgements

Thanks to Karen and Bruce Bellenir, Maria Franklin, Joan Margeson and Jenifer Swanson for their help with the many details involved in the making of this sourcebook. This book is dedicated to Mary Ann Klaudt ("Great Grandma Mary"), whose 97 years of healthy living are an inspiration to my daughters and me.

Note from the Editor

This book is part of Omnigraphics' *Health Reference Series*. The series provides basic information about a broad range of medical concerns. It is not intended to serve as a tool for diagnosing illness, in prescribing treatments, or as a substitute for the physician/patient relationship. All persons concerned about medical symptoms or the possibility of disease are encouraged to seek professional care from an appropriate health care provider.

Our Advisory Board

The *Health Reference Series* is reviewed by an Advisory Board comprised of librarians from public, academic, and medical libraries. We would like to thank the following board members for providing guidance to the development of this series:

Dr. Lynda Baker,
Associate Professor of Library and Information Science,
Wayne State University, Detroit, MI

Nancy Bulgarelli,
William Beaumont Hospital Library, Royal Oak, MI

Karen Imarasio,
Bloomfield Township Public Library, Bloomfield Township, MI

Karen Morgan,
Mardigian Library, University of Michigan-Dearborn,
Dearborn, MI

Rosemary Orlando,
St. Clair Shores Public Library, St. Clair Shores, MI

Health Reference Series *Update Policy*

The inaugural book in the *Health Reference Series* was the first edition of *Cancer Sourcebook* published in 1992. Since then, the *Series* has been enthusiastically received by librarians and in the medical community. In order to maintain the standard of providing high-quality health information for the lay person, the editorial staff at Omnigraphics felt it was necessary to implement a policy of updating volumes when warranted.

Medical researchers have been making tremendous strides, and it is the purpose of the *Health Reference Series* to stay current with the most recent advances. Each decision to update a volume will be made on an individual basis. Some of the considerations will include how much new information is available and the feedback we receive from people who use the books. If there is a topic you would like to see added to the update list, or an area of medical concern you feel has not been adequately addressed, please write to:

Editor
Health Reference Series
Omnigraphics, Inc.
615 Griswold
Detroit, MI 48226

The commitment to providing on-going coverage of important medical developments has also led to some format changes in the *Health Reference Series*. Beginning with books published in 1999, each new volume will be individually titled and called a "First Edition." Subsequent updates will carry sequential edition numbers. To help avoid confusion and to provide maximum flexibility in our ability to respond to informational needs, the practice of consecutively numbering each volume has been discontinued.

Part One

Introduction to Women and Heart Disease

Chapter 1

Women and Heart Disease: The Statistics

Heart disease. Traditionally thought of as a man's disease, many women tend not to give it much thought. "It could never happen to me," some women say. Unfortunately, their thinking is wrong. Sometimes....dead wrong.

The Numbers Are Revealing

Each year, heart attacks claim the lives of nearly 500,000 men and women in the United States. Almost half of the fatal heart attacks, about 240,000, are sustained by women. Another 88,000 women die each year from stroke. On a larger scale, all heart and blood vessel disease combined claim more than 485,000 women's lives annually. By comparison, less than 223,000 women perish each year from all forms of cancer.

Just like for men, heart disease is the leading cause of death for women. Surprisingly, a woman is also less likely to survive a heart attack than a man.

Heart Attack: What Is It?

A heart attack occurs when the supply of blood to part of the heart muscle itself is closed off completely. It happens because one or more of the coronary arteries that supplies blood to the heart is blocked.

This is usually caused by a blood clot. Depending on how long the supply is cut off, the muscle cells in that area of the heart may suffer permanent damage or die.

Heart attacks result from blood vessel disease in the heart, called coronary artery disease. Diseases of the heart and blood vessels are known as cardiovascular diseases. Other major heart or vascular diseases include stroke (brain attack), rheumatic heart disease and hypertension (high blood pressure).

Heart Attack: Know the Warning Signs

You've probably heard about the typical heart attack warning signs. It's classically described like a "heavy object sitting on your chest." A key warning sign is a pain traveling down the left arm.

These symptoms, however, are typical for middle-aged men and not necessarily for women. According to a number of physicians, women are more likely to have the following symptoms:

- vague abdominal discomfort
- nausea and vomiting
- fatigue
- shortness of breath (trouble catching your breath)
- arm and/or chest pain

It is important that you call 911 if you experience these symptoms, or recognize them in someone else. The sooner you take actions with heart attack warning signs, the better your chances of reducing permanent heart muscle damage or even death.

Facts about Women and Heart Disease

- One in nine women aged 45 to 64 has some form of cardiovascular disease.

- One in three women over age 65 has some form of cardiovascular disease.

- About 6,000 women under the age of 65 die each year of heart attack.

- Women show signs and symptoms for heart disease approximately 10 years later than men.

- Forty percent of the heart attacks in women are fatal.

- Heart attack death rates for African-American women are 1.4 times that of white women.

- High blood pressure affects one in three African-American women.

(Source for these statistics: American Heart Association/Framingham Study)

Source: *"Women and Heart Disease: The Statistics are Startling,"* (Brochure). Kettering Medical Center, Dayton, OH. (Information in this brochure was printed in cooperation with the American Heart Association)

Chapter 2

The Facts about Heart Disease and Women: Are You at Risk?

Heart disease is a woman's concern. Every woman's concern. One in ten American women 45 to 64 years of age has some form of heart disease, and this increases to one in four women over 65. Heart disease is the number one killer of American women. In addition, 2 million women have had a stroke, and 93,000 women die of stroke each year.

This chapter tells you what kinds of habits and health conditions increase the chances of developing these diseases—and what you can do to keep your heart healthy.

What Are These Diseases?

Both heart disease and stroke are known as cardiovascular diseases, which are disorders of the heart and blood vessel system. Coronary heart disease is a disease of the blood vessels of the heart, known as "coronary arteries." Coronary heart disease causes chest pain (angina) and heart attacks. Blood brings oxygen and nutrients to the heart. When too little blood flows to the heart, angina results. When the blood flow is critically reduced, a heart attack occurs. A lack of blood flow to the brain or, in some cases, bleeding in the brain causes a stroke. Some other cardiovascular diseases are high blood pressure and rheumatic heart disease.

Exerpted from *Heart Healthy Handbook for Women*, National Heart, Lung, and Blood Institute (NHLBI), NIH Publication No. 98-3654, revised August 1998.

Who Gets Cardiovascular Diseases?

Some women have more "risk factors" for cardiovascular diseases than others. Risk factors are habits or traits that make a person more likely to develop a disease. Some risk factors for heart-related problems cannot be changed, but many others can be.

The major risk factors for cardiovascular disease that you can do something about are cigarette smoking, high blood pressure, high blood cholesterol, overweight, and physical inactivity. Other risk factors, such as diabetes, also are conditions you have some control over. Even just one risk factor will raise your chances of having heart-related problems. But the more risk factors you have, the more likely you are to develop cardiovascular diseases—and the more concerned you should be about protecting your heart health.

Heart Disease Risk Factors

Risk factors are habits or traits that make a person more likely to develop a disease. Many of those for heart disease can be controlled. These include:

- Cigarette smoking
- High blood pressure
- High blood cholesterol
- Overweight
- Physical inactivity
- Diabetes

Other risk factors include:

- Stress
- Birth Control Pills
- Alcohol Consumption
- Hormones and Menopause

The more risk factors you have, the greater your risk. So take action—take control!

For More Information

If you would like to know more about keeping your heart healthy, the National Heart, Lung, and Blood Institute (NHLBI) has available free fact sheets on these subjects: preventing and controlling high blood pressure, preventing and controlling high blood cholesterol, quitting smoking, the heart benefits of physical activity, and hormone replacement therapy (HRT).

Contact:

NHLBI Information Center
P.O. Box 30105
Bethesda, MD 20824-0105
Phone: (301) 251-1222
Fax: (301) 251-1223
Or check out the NHLBI web site at http://www.nhlbi.nih.gov/nhlbi/nhlbi.htm.

U.S. Department of Health And Human Services
Public Health Service
National Institutes of Health
National Heart, Lung, and Blood Institute

Chapter 3

Coronary Disease in Women: The Leading Killer

Coronary heart disease in women is often diagnosed later and treated less aggressively than in men. The first step toward better care is to understand what's different about women's coronary risk factors, symptoms, and responses to testing and treatment.

Coronary heart disease (CHD) is the number one killer of American women. Of the nearly 500,000 fatal myocardial infarctions (MIs) that occur each year, more than 233,000 strike women.[1] In addition, women have slimmer chances than men of surviving a heart attack long term.

One in three women aged 65 or older and 1 in 9 women aged 45-64 will develop clinical evidence of CHD.[2] Yet many women and some physicians still do not recognize CHD as a serious health risk to women. According to a 1995 Gallup survey:

- 80% of 505 women aged 45-75 and 32% of 300 primary care physicians surveyed did not know that heart disease is the leading cause of death among women.

- 88% of physicians and 70% of women believed that the signs and symptoms of heart disease are the same in women and men. In fact, women's symptoms may differ from those typically seen in men.

"Coronary Disease: The Leading Killer," by Charles H. Hennekens, Debra Ruth Judelson, and Nanette K. Wenger, in *Patient Care*, August 15, 1996, Vol. 30, No. 13, (Women's Heart Health, Special Issue) Pg. 116(12), © 1996 Medical Economics Publishing; reprinted with permission.

- 67% of physicians believed there is no difference in CHD risk factors for women and men.

- 89% of primary care physicians stated that physicians need more education about CHD in women.

Another survey of 337 women posed the question, What illness do you fear the most?[3] Three times as many women feared breast cancer as feared heart disease. Nearly three fourths (73%) of the women perceived their risk of developing heart disease by age 70 as less than 1%. Only 25% considered the cardioprotective effects of estrogen in their decision to begin hormone replacement.

CHD and MI are often underdiagnosed in women. A principal reason is that women are less likely than men to associate their symptoms with heart disease and are more likely to wait longer after the onset of chest pain before seeking medical help. In addition, gender bias remains a significant issue among physicians who evaluate women for symptoms of chest pain, although major favorable changes have occurred in recent years.

The primary care physician has an important role to play in the prevention, diagnosis, and treatment of CHD in women. The first goal is education—sending the message to women that they are vulnerable to heart disease and that their risk increases dramatically after menopause. A woman has to know the symptoms of CHD and MI so that she will not hesitate to seek evaluation for potentially heart-related chest discomfort, fatigue, and weakness.

Your role includes assessing her risk factors, screening throughout her life for development of high blood pressure and lipid abnormalities, and counseling her on risk modification strategies and preventive therapies. Together, these interventions can significantly reduce the impact of CHD.

Risk Factors in Women

Women and men share many of the same risk factors for CHD, but the degree of risk often differs. The patterns of risk may also vary with age. A man's risk of heart attack typically begins to increase at age 40-45. A woman's risk starts to rise sharply about 10 years later— after menopause at about age 50-55. Women ultimately catch up with men, as the CHD risk continues to rise among women in their 70s and 80s. Women tend to be 10-15 years older than men when they first present with symptomatic CHD, and this may partly account for their higher death rates.

Hypertension

After age 65, more women than men have hypertension, and it is more likely to cause CHD complications in women. In men, systolic blood pressure peaks in middle age; in women, it can continue to rise until at least age 80. Isolated systolic hypertension—a result of decreased arterial elasticity—is more common among women than men and affects approximately 30% of women older than 65. Both combined systolic/diastolic hypertension and isolated systolic hypertension are associated with an increased risk of CHD as well as stroke.

In the United States, hypertension affects 51% of white women and 79% of black women older than 45.[2] The disorder is not only more prevalent, but also more severe, in black women and may be explained at least in part by obesity.

Lifestyle changes to reduce blood pressure include weight control, regular physical activity, and reduced sodium and alcohol consumption. According to an analysis of 17 trials, drug therapy to reduce mild to moderate elevations in diastolic blood pressure can reduce the risk of CHD by about 16% and stroke by 38%.[4]

Cigarette Smoking

The risk of CHD is 2-4 times higher in women who smoke 20 or more cigarettes per day (heavy smokers) than in female nonsmokers, regardless of menopausal status. Furthermore, smoking lowers the age when menopause occurs by an average of 2-6 years, widening the window of increased CHD risk. In the Nurses' Health Study, even women who were light smokers (1-4 cigarettes per day) had at least twice the risk of CHD as nonsmokers.

Cigarettes that claim reduced tar, nicotine, and carbon monoxide content apparently do not pose a lower CHD risk. Smoking presents an even greater danger for women who are already at high risk for CHD because of a combination of older age, family history of CHD, overweight, and other risk factors. The risk of MI among smokers older than 35 who use high-dose oral contraceptives (OCs) is about 40 times higher than the risk in nonsmokers who don't use OCs.

Men who smoke have their first heart attack an average of seven years earlier than male nonsmokers. In sharp contrast, women who smoke have their first heart attack 19 years earlier than nonsmoking women. Although the number of men and women smokers has declined steadily over the past 35 years, women smokers have been taking up the habit earlier and smoking more. Women patients should know that the risk of CHD begins to fall within months after they stop smoking and decreases to that of a nonsmoker within 3-5 years.

Obesity

Nearly 50% of black women, 48% of Mexican American women, and more than 32% of white women are 20% or more above their desirable weight. The risk of CHD is tripled in these women, and even those who are moderately overweight may have twice the risk of lean women. In fact, a linear relationship exists between body weight and both cardiovascular and total mortality.

Abdominal and upper body obesity further increase a woman's risk, and the risk rises dramatically among those who have a waist-to-hip ratio greater than 0.8. Women tend to gain weight after age 35, and even moderate weight gain that puts a woman's weight at the high end of the normal range increases CHD risk.[5]

Age, Race, and Family History

Advancing age increases the risk of CHD in both women and men. Having a family member who had CHD or an MI at a young age be-fore 55 for men and before 65 for women—is a risk factor for CHD. If the relative was a woman, the risk is even greater for both men and women. Blacks have a greater risk of CHD, primarily because of higher average blood pressure levels. Between the ages of 35 and 74, black women are 1.5 times more likely to die of an MI than are white women, and they have three times the coronary death rate of women of other races.

Diabetes Mellitus

In people older than 45, women are twice as likely as men to de-velop diabetes. Diabetes is also a more potent risk factor for CHD in women than men. Diabetes increases the risk of heart disease by 2-3 times in men, but it raises the risk in women by 3-7 times, thereby negating the gender advantage that women have for developing CHD. This increased risk is present even among premenopausal women. Diabetes also heightens the effects of other CHD risk factors. It is more prevalent among black than among white Americans, and in women, diabetes-related mortality is twice as high in blacks as in whites. Current data are insufficient to determine whether strict con-trol of blood glucose levels reduces CHD risk.

14

At all levels of body weight, obesity is the major risk factor for adult-onset diabetes. The incidence of diabetes can be reduced by regular exercise.

Lipid Profile

During much of their adult lives, women have a healthier lipid profile than men, with higher levels of high-density lipoprotein (HDL) cholesterol and lower levels of low-density lipo-protein (LDL) cholesterol. With advancing age, a woman's total cholesterol level begins to rise, mostly due to increases in LDL cholesterol, which can continue to rise until a woman is well into her 70s. At older ages, LDL cholesterol levels in women are higher, on average, than in men. Just as in men, the data suggest that interventions to lower LDL cholesterol and raise HDL cholesterol reduce a woman's risk of CHD. A woman's HDL cholesterol level is an average of 10 points higher than a man's, and some have suggested that national guidelines for HDL cholesterol levels should be set higher for women.

In men, the LDL cholesterol level appears to be the most important risk factor for CHD, with HDL cholesterol ranked second and the triglyceride level third. Triglycerides contribute to CHD by making LDL more atherogenic. In women, HDL cholesterol seems to be the most important risk factor, though some would question this. Elevated triglyceride levels may be associated with an increase in CHD and acute coronary events in women, especially when associated with low HDL levels.

Menopause

Menopause, whether natural or surgical, is the CHD risk factor unique to women. In natural menopause, a woman's estrogen levels decrease over the course of several years, and, therefore, her risk of CHD begins to increase somewhat even before she actually stops menstruating. Estrogen may protect against CHD through its effects on cholesterol levels, clotting factors, the vasculature, and endothelial—and possibly myocardial function. Estrogen increases HDL cholesterol levels and decreases LDL cholesterol levels, lowers fibrinogen levels, is a weak antioxidant, and has some calcium channel blocking activity. Estrogen is also a vasodilator and can cause even atherosclerotic arteries to dilate in response to appropriate stimuli by normalizing endothelial function.

Estrogen may also stabilize atherosclerotic lesions. Recent research suggests that MI is caused by unstable atheromatous lesions that contain a sizable lipid core. These lesions may cause only 40-70% arterial narrowing but are more predictive of MI because they are more likely to rupture. Older plaques that cause 80-90% narrowing of a vessel may lead to exertional angina but are more stable and not as likely to rupture and cause an MI.

Estrogen may modify factors that convert a stable to an unstable lesion. Loss of estrogen at menopause may destabilize the lipid core, prompting vasospasm, clot formation, and a subsequent acute ischemic event.

Other Risk Factors

Heavy alcohol consumption is a risk factor for CHD. Although low to moderate daily alcohol consumption may offer the same cardioprotective effect in women as it does in men—about a 40% reduced risk of CHD when compared to nondrinkers—the deleterious effects of alcohol preclude any recommendations for nondrinking women to start. In addition, women who drink alcohol may be at increased risk of breast cancer.

Physical inactivity also increases a woman's risk of CHD. Women who engage in regular physical activity have a 50-75% reduced risk of CHD when compared to inactive women. One case control study of postmenopausal women found that leisure time physical activity with modest energy expenditure decreased the risk of MI by about 50%.[6] Walking for exercise for about 45 minutes three times a week was sufficient to reduce MI risk, and more strenuous activity did not further decrease the risk.

Strategies for Prevention

At the outset, women have to understand that they are vulnerable to heart disease. Each woman should know her own risk profile and understand how to act on it. The main objective of any CHD prevention strategy is to reduce and, if possible, eliminate the significant risk factors. She won't be able to change her genetic propensity for CHD, but she can stop smoking, control blood pressure, lose weight, exercise, or modify other risk factors.

Obvious Places to Start

Smoking cessation is crucial—cigarette smoking is a major preventable risk factor for CHD in women. Physical activity has a direct beneficial effect on the heart and also improves other coronary risk factors, including body weight, lipid profile, and diabetes control. Other obvious preventive measures include controlling high blood pressure and following a prudent diet.

Antioxidants

Basic research has demonstrated that vitamin E and other antioxidant vitamins inhibit either the oxidation of LDL cholesterol or its uptake into the endothelium of coronary arteries. Dietary antioxidants represent a promising means of decreasing CHD risk, but reliable evidence from randomized trials in women is required before any rational clinical and policy decisions can be made. Such data are accumulating in ongoing large-scale trials in women, including the Women's Health Study of 40,000 apparently healthy female health professionals aged 45 or older.

Aspirin

Both men and women who are having an MI, have survived an occlusive cardiovascular event, or have well-established CHD benefit from aspirin therapy. Large prevention trials have demonstrated a 40% reduction in first MIs among men who were randomly assigned to low-dose aspirin, but no such prospective primary prevention trial data are yet available for women. The Women's Health Study will assess the effects of low-dose aspirin, as well as of vitamin E. Currently, the use of aspirin in this context represents an individual clinical decision made by the physician and patient. The decision must weigh the benefit of reducing the risk profile versus the possible side effects of long-term administration.

Hormone Replacement Therapy

Although data are not yet available from randomized trials, women who self-select for postmenopausal hormone replacement therapy (HRT) have a reduced risk of coronary events of as much as 50% in observational studies. In addition to alleviation of menopausal symptoms and decreased risk of osteoporosis, the cardioprotective effects of HRT after either natural or surgical menopause may be a consideration in the decision to begin HRT. Two ongoing randomized trials are evaluating HRT in women with and without heart disease: the Heart and Estrogen/Progestin Replacement Study (HERS) and the

Women's Health Initiative. It should be emphasized that most studies to date have used unopposed oral estrogen therapy and that no data are available as yet on the cardiovascular benefits of the estrogen patch.

Estrogen's negative effects include a modest increase in triglyceride levels, an increase in gallbladder disease, and worsening of migraine headaches. In addition to increasing the size of uterine fibroids, the most serious adverse effects of estrogen therapy are on the endometrium and breast. In the Post-menopausal Estrogen and Progestin Interventions (PEPI) Trial, unopposed estrogen caused a 33% three-year incidence of endometrial hyperplasia, which precludes the use of estrogen alone except in women who have had a hysterectomy.

The addition of progestin to the regimen protects the endometrium from estrogen's proliferative effects. Furthermore, the combination of estrogen with various progestins appears to have cardioprotective effects on coronary risk factors that are only slightly less than those of estrogen alone. Estrogenprogestin combinations increase HDL cholesterol levels, although to a lesser degree than estrogen alone. They also decrease LDL cholesterol, fibrinogen, and plasminogen activator inhibitor levels, all of which rise after menopause. Natural progesterone seems to interfere least with estrogen's cardioprotective effects. Few or no studies have examined HRT's effect on actual coronary events.

The risk of breast cancer is the concern raised most often by women contemplating estrogen replacement or HRT. The Nurses' Health Study data suggest that using estrogen for more than five years may increase a woman's risk of breast cancer by 40-50%, although definitive long-term data are not yet available. Other studies have shown no increased risk, whereas aggregates of multiple studies reveal an increased risk of about 10%. These conflicting findings make it difficult to establish a benefit/risk ratio for HRT. Consequently, each patient must weigh her risk factors for breast cancer and CHD. It's revealing, however, that even a postmenopausal woman who is diagnosed with nonmetastatic breast cancer is more likely to die of CHD.

New research on different types of estrogen may help resolve the HRT dilemma. Some natural plant estrogens, such as those found in soy products, are selective estrogen receptor modulators. They appear to have a positive effect on bone, may benefit the heart, and do not seem to have an effect on the breast or uterus.

How estrogen replacement therapy may protect the heart:

- Increases high-density lipoprotein cholesterol
- Decreases low-density lipoprotein (LDL) cholesterol

- Reduces oxidation of LDL cholesterol
- Lowers uptake of LDL cholesterol in blood vessels
- Decreases lipoprotein
- Binds to vascular estrogen receptors
- Reduces vascular tone
- Preserves endothelial function
- Increases prostaglandin 12 release
- Decreases thromboxane [A.sub.2] formation
- Decreases fibrinogen
- Reduces plasminogen activator inhibitor
- Decreases fasting blood glucose and insulin levels

Adapted with permission from Sullivan JM: Coronary arteriography in estrogen treated postmenopausal women. *Prog Cardiovasc Dis* 1995;38:211 222.

CHD and Angina: A Different Picture in Women?

Women with myocardial ischemia may not experience chest pain on exertion. This is particularly true of older women with a sedentary lifestyle. Common anginal equivalents in women may include the following:

- A feeling of shortness of breath with or without exertion

- Pressure or discomfort in the chest that comes and goes with or without exertion

- Chronic fatigue, inability to complete normal activities, and bouts of nausea that seem unrelated to diet.

Rather than asking the patient whether she has had chest pain, using words such as pressure, heaviness, and discomfort to ask about her symptoms might better help to identify CHD. An initial evaluation should concentrate on ruling out noncardiac causes of chest pain, including esophageal spasm and reflux, costochondritis, musculoskeletal symptoms that cause heaviness and tightness in the chest wall, hyperventilation due to anxiety, and nonischemic cardiac symptoms. Patients whose symptoms suggest angina require further evaluation.

There is disagreement on the reliability of the exercise ECG in women. Some authorities claim that exercise testing has comparable rates of false-positive results in women and men if the resting ECG is normal. Others, however, believe the false-positive rate may be as much as 40% higher in women, even with a normal resting ECG. What's clear is that women are more likely to have abnormal resting ECGs, and, in this group, exercise testing is unwise. Also consider the pretest probability of false-positive results in premenopausal women who do not have a number of risk factors for CHD.

Exercise nuclear perfusion studies have low false-positive rates in women when correction for breast attenuation is made. Exercise and pharmacologic echocardiography can identify wall motion abnormalities and may be valuable for detecting single-vessel disease. This is important because single-vessel disease is relatively more common in women. Newer tests, such as positron emission tomography (PET) and MRI, are under investigation for women.

As recently as 10-15 years ago, 10 times as many men as women (40% versus 4%) were referred for angiography following an abnormal result on a noninvasive test, such as myocardial perfusion imaging. This pattern has changed dramatically, and men are now only twice as likely to have a more aggressive evaluation in this situation.

Different Treatment Options?

Since CHD differs somewhat in women and men, researchers are turning their attention to the subtleties of prevention, detection, and treatment of heart disease in women. In general, men may be overtested and overtreated, and women previously tended to be undertested and undertreated. Some reluctance to treat women aggressively, particularly with surgery, stems from the observation that women fare more poorly than men following procedures such as angioplasty and coronary artery bypass grafting.

This has several possible explanations:

- Women tend to be older and have more comorbidity when they undergo treatment.

- They tend to defer evaluation and treatment and present with more advanced and often unstable disease, requiring urgent intervention.

- A woman's arteries are typically smaller in diameter than a man's.

- The catheters and other instruments and procedures used in newer angioplasty procedures may be too large for use in women.

Several advances have been made. The trends toward earlier diagnosis of CHD, earlier intervention, and less emergency treatment are hopeful signs. Smaller catheter-based devices may enhance the success of invasive procedures in women, although no sex-specific data on the efficacy of stents are yet available. A key point: Although women may not fare as well as men after angioplasty or bypass surgery, they still do better than women who are candidates for these procedures but do not have them.

Many drugs to treat CHD or MI have received limited assessment in women. Although some drugs that are used to treat CHD in men appear to be equally beneficial in women, the correct dosing for them is still uncertain. Because of their smaller body mass, some women may need lower dosages. Undermedication continues to be a problem for women. According to one recent study of patients with acute MI who were candidates for treatment with aspirin, thrombolytic agents, and B-blockers, drug use was consistently lower for women than for men (odds ratios for women: 0.7, 0.7, and 0.9, respectively).[7]

—Prepared by Vicki Glaser, Contributing Editor

References

1. American Heart Association: *Heart and Stroke Facts: 1996 Statiststical Supplement.* Dallas, American Heart Association, 1995, p 9.

2. Wenger NK: Coronary heart disease in women: The high prevalence of coronary risk factors and the importance of prevention. *J Med Assoc Ga* 1995; 84:323-328.

3. Pilote L, Hlatky MA: Attitudes of women toward hormone therapy and prevention of heart disease. *Arp Heart J* 1995; 129:1237-1238.

4. Hebert PR, Moser M, Mayer J, Hennekens CH: Recent evidence on drug therapy of mild to moderate hypertension and decreased risk of coronary heart disease. *Arch Intern Med* 1993; 153:578-581.

5. Willett WC, Manson JE, Stampfer MJ, et al: Weight, weight change, and coronary heart disease in women: Risk within the "normal" weight range. *JAMA* 1995; 273:461-465.

6. Lemaitre RN, Heckbert SR, Psaty BM, et al: Leisure-time physical activity and the risk of nonfatal myocardial infarction

in postmenopausal women. *Arch Intern Med* 1995; 155:2302-2308.

7. McLaughlin T J, Soumerai SB, Willison DJ, et al: Adherence to national guidelines for drug treatment of suspected acute myocardial infarction: Evidence for undertreatment in women and the elderly. *Arch Intern Med* 1996; 156:799-805.

8. Dorr AE, Gundersen K, Schneider JC Jr, et al: Colestipol hydrochloride in hypercholesterolemic patients—effect on serum cholesterol and mortality. *J Chronic Ois* 1978; 31:5-14.

9. Frantz ID Jr, Dawson EA, Ashman PL, et al: Test of effect of lipid lowering by diet on cardiovascular risk: The Minnesota Coronary Survey. *Arteriosclerosis* 1989; 9:129-135.

10. SHEP Cooperative Research Group: Prevention of stroke by antihypertensive drug treatment in older persons with isolated systolic hypertension: Final results of the Systolic Hypertension in the Elderly Program (SHEP). *JAMA* 1991; 265:3255-3264.

11. Stampfer MJ, Colditz GA: Estrogen replacement therapy and coronary heart disease: Quantitative assessment of the epidemiologic evidence. *Prey Med* 1991; 20:47-63.

12. The Writing Group for the PEPI Trial: Effects of estrogen or estrogen/progestin regimens on heart disease risk factors in postmenopausal women: The Post-menopausal Estrogen/Progestin Interventions (PEPI) Trial. *JAMA* 1995; 273:199-208.

Suggested Reading

Allen JK, Blumenthal RS: Coronary risk factors in women six months after coronary artery bypass grafting. *Am J Cardiol* 1995; 75:1092-1095.

Cannistra LB, O'Malley CJ, Balady G J: Comparison of outcome of cardiac rehabilitation in black women and white women. *Am J Cardiol* 1995; 75:890-893.

Clark LT, Karve MM, Rones KT, et al: Obesity, distribution of body fat and coronary artery disease in black women. *Am J Cardiol* 1994; 73:895-896.

Douglas PS, Ginsburg GS: The evaluation of chest pain in women. *N Engl J Med* 1996; 334:1311-1315.

Grodstein F, Stampfer M: The epidemiology of coronary heart disease and estrogen replacement in postmenopausal women. *Prog Cardiovasc Dis* 1995; 38:199-210.

Johnson PA, Goldman L, Cray EJ, et al: Gender differences in the management of acute chest pain: Support for the "Yentl syndrome." *J Gen Intern Med* 1996; 11:209-217.

Judelson DR: Coronary heart disease in women: Risk factors and prevention. *J Am Med Wom Assoc* 1994; 49;186-191,197.

Kushi LH, Folsom AR, Prineas RJ, et al: Dietary antioxidant vitamins and death from coronary heart disease in postmenopausal women. *N Engl J Med* 1996; 334:1156-1162.

Lehmann JB, Wehner PS, Lehmann CU, et al: Gender bias in the evaluation of chest pain in the emergency department. *Am J Cardiol* 1996; 77:641-644.

Manson JE, Lea IM: Exercise for women: How much pain for optimal gain? editorial. *N Engl J Med* 1996; 334:1325-1327.

Marwick TH, Anderson T, Williams MJ, et al: Exercise echocardiography is an accurate and cost-efficient technique for detection of coronary artery disease in women. *J Am Coll Cardiol* 1995; 26:335-341.

Muller JE, Abela GS, Nesto RW, et al: Triggers, acute risk factors and vulnerable plaques: The lexicon of a new frontier. *J Am Coll Cardiol* 1994; 23:809-813.

Murabito JM: Women and cardiovascalar disease: Contributions from the Framingham Heart Study. *J Am Med Wom Assoc* 1995; 50:35-39,55.

Psaty BM, Heckbert SR, Atkins D, et al: The risk of myocardial infarction associated with the combined use of estrogens and progestins in postmenopausal women. *Arch Intern Med* 1994; 154:1333-1339.

Rich-Edwards JW, Manson JE, Hennekens CH, et al: The primary prevention of coronary heart disease in women. *N Engl J Med* 1995; 332:1758-1766.

Simkin-Silverman L, Wing RR, Hansen DH, et al: Prevention of cardiovascular risk factor elevations in healthy premenopausal women. *Prev Med* 1995; 24:509-517.

Sullivan JM: Coronary arteriography in estrogen-treated postmenopausal women. *Prog Cardiovasc Dis* 1995; 38:211-222.

Volterrani M, Rosano G, Coats A, et al: Estrogen acutely increases peripheral blood flow in postmenopausal women. *Am J Med* 1995; 99:119-122.

Walsh JM, Grady D: Treatment of hyperlipidemia in women. *JAMA* 1995; 274:1152-1158.

Wenger NK: A symposium: Gender differences in cardiac imaging, editorial. *Am J Cardiac Imaging* 1996; 10:42-43.

Williams PT: High-density lipoprotein cholesterol and other risk factors for coronary heart disease in female runners. *N Engl J Med* 1996; 334:1298-1303.

Women at Risk for Hypertension

Nearly half of the more than 50 million Americans who have high blood pressure are women. In 90-95% of cases of hypertension, the cause is not known. Men are at greater risk for high blood pressure than women until age 55. Between ages 55-74, the risks for developing hypertension are about equal in men and women. After age 74, women are at greater risk than men. After menopause, a woman's blood pressure often rises and may continue to increase well into her 80s. In 1992, women accounted for 58% of all deaths attributable to high blood pressure.[1]

Women taking oral contraceptives (OCs) tend to have blood pressures that are about 2-3 mmhg higher than in women who don't take OCs. Regarding the risk of coronary disease however, the risk of using OCs is small in comparison with the risk posed by cigarette smoking, but there is a clear and alarming synergy between them.

Black women have a much higher risk of hypertension than white women, and the disease tends to develop at an earlier age and to be more severe. Of all deaths in black women in this country, 21.2% are attributable to hypertension, compared to 4.8% among white women.

Other risk factors for hypertension include obesity, menopause, a family history of high blood pressure, and pregnancy, with the greatest risk during the third trimester. Recent studies suggest that women obtain the same benefit from lifestyle interventions and drug therapies as men do and that hypertension should be treated aggressively in women of all ages, as it is in men. Women may be more sensitive than men to some antihypertensive drugs, such as [Beta]-blockers, and may need lower dosages to achieve the same reduction in blood pressure without side effects.

1. American Heart Association: *Heart and Stroke Facts: 1996 Statistical Supplement*. Dallas, American Heart Association, 1995, p 12.

Is Thrombolytic Therapy Appropriate in Women?

Women and men with acute myocardial infarction (MI) benefit equally from thrombolysis with agents such as streptokinase (Streptase) or alteplase (Activase), but women have more bleeding complications, including hemorrhagic stroke.[1] More women than men are ineligible for thrombolytic therapy because they tend to delay coming to the hospital until it is too late. In a study that compared six-week incidences of death and reinfarction in women and men with MI who were eligible for thrombolytic therapy, women's higher rates were largely attributable to their older age and higher incidence of diabetes.[2]

The use of thrombolytic therapy is not contraindicated in women who are menstruating or are immediately postpartum. Neither of these states appears to increase the risk of severe bleeding, stroke, or poorer clinical outcome.

1. Lincoff AM, Califf RM, Ellis SG, et al: Thrombolytic therapy for women with myocardial infarction: Is there a gender gap? *J Am Coll Cardiol* 1993; 22:1780-1787.

2. Becker RC, Terrin M, Ross R, et al: Comparison of clinical outcomes for women and men after acute myocardial infarction. *Am Intern Med* 1994; 120:638-645.

Article Consultants

Charles H. Hennekens, MD, DrPH, and Eugene Braunwald are Professor of Medicine and Professor of Ambulatory Care and Prevention, Harvard Medical School; and Chief, Division of Preventive Medicine, Brigham and Women's Hospital, Boston.

Debra Ruth Judelson, MD, is a Senior Partner with Cardiovascular Medical Group of Southern California, Beverly Hills; and Consultant, Cedars-Sinai Medical Center, Los Angeles. She is Chair of the

Committee on Cardiovascular Disease in Women and President-elect of the American Medical Women's Association.

Nanette K. Wenger, MD, is Professor of Medicine, Division of Cardiology, Emory University School of Medicine; Consultant, Emory Heart Center; and Director, Cardiac Clinics, Grady Memorial Hospital, Atlanta.

Chapter 4

A Woman's Heart

Many women experience more severe first heart attacks than men. When it comes to matters of the heart, women are often thought to be more profoundly affected than men. It's no different, it seems, with diseases of the heart. Coronary heart disease is the leading cause of death for women in America and most developed countries.

Although the overall death rate for heart disease has declined in the United States over the last several decades, the rate of decline has been less for women than for men. In fact, the number of deaths due to heart disease among women has been increasing. With more women living longer and nearly twice as many U.S. women dying from heart disease and stroke than all forms of cancer combined (including breast cancer), heart disease in women certainly is a major health issue.

New research confirms that women may fare worse than men following a first heart attack. A study in the October 28, 1998, issue of *JAMA* found that women are at greater risk of death within the first month after their first heart attack and also are at greater risk of death or requiring readmission to a hospital within six months than men. The researchers found that the reason women had more than a 70% greater risk of death than men after a first heart attack may be due to the more severe nature and complications associated with women's heart attacks. The difference between men and women existed

JAMA, *The Journal of the American Medical Association*, Oct. 28, 1998, Vol. 280, No. 16, Pg. 1462(1), © 1998 American Medical Association; reprinted with permission.

regardless of the women's ages or their other risk factors for heart disease. Heart disease also is more likely to go undetected in women than men. Women need to learn more about heart disease and ways to prevent it.

Risk Factors for Heart Disease

- Cigarette smoking
- High blood pressure
- High cholesterol
- Diabetes
- Family history of heart disease
- Obesity
- Inactivity
- African American women are at higher risk than other women in the United States

Role Menopause Plays

A woman's risk of heart disease increases as she approaches menopause and continues to increase as she ages. Studies have shown that postmenopausal women have higher levels of blood lipids and cholesterol, which are risk factors for heart disease. Researchers believe the changes in women's bodies may be due to a combination of aging, weight gain, and the effects of menopause itself, including reduced levels of the hormone estrogen.

How to Protect Against Heart Disease

- Don't smoke
- Get regular exercise and maintain healthy body weight
- Eat a diet low in saturated fat and high in fruits, vegetables, whole grains, and fiber
- Avoid heavy drinking, which can raise cholesterol levels and blood pressure
- Get treatment for high blood pressure or diabetes
- Talk to your doctor about hormone replacement therapy after menopause

For More Information

American Heart Association
National Heart, Lung, and Blood Institute
NHLBI Information Center
P.O. Box 30105
Bethesda, MD 20824-0105
(888) MY-HEART
Internet: http://www.nhlbi.nih.gov *or*
http://www.women.americanheart.org

Chapter 5

Women's Heart and Stroke Quiz

Heart disease and stroke are responsible for 40% of all female deaths in Canada. Do you know whether your medical history or lifestyle is putting you at risk? Are you ready to take charge and reduce your risk? Take the Heart and Stroke Foundation's Women's Heart and Stroke Quiz and find out how you score.

Are You at Risk? Your Personal Medical Risk Profile.

1. Has your father, mother, sister(s) or brother(s) suffered a heart attack, required heart surgery, or had a stroke prior to age 65?

    a) Yes   b) No

2. Are you diabetic?

    a) Yes   b) No

3. Have you been told by a health professional that you have high blood pressure or do you take medication to lower your blood pressure?

    a) Yes   b) No

Chatelaine, September 1996, Vol. 69, No.9, Pg. 2(3), © 1996 MacLean Hunter Ltd. (Canada), developed by the Heart and Stroke Foundation of Ontario; reprinted with permission.

4. Have you been told by a health professional that you have high cholesterol or have you ever been prescribed a cholesterol-lowering medication?

   a) Yes   b) No

5. Has your doctor told you that you have a heart condition, have you ever suffered a heart attack, required heart surgery, or had a stroke?

   a) Yes   b) No

6. Are you:

   a) Age 65 or over   b) Age 40 - 65 years   c) Under age 40

How Healthy Is Your Lifestyle?

1. Do you smoke?

   a) Yes—heavily (one or more packs a day)

   b) Yes—(less than one pack a day)

   c) Not now—(quit within the past three years)

   d) Never smoked or quit more than three years ago

2. Do you live or work with people who smoke?

   a) Yes   b) No

3. Do you perform physical activity (such as walking, jogging, cycling, swimming, step-training or dancing) for a daily total of 30 minutes, three or more times each week?

   a) No   b) Yes

4. How would you describe the amount of fat in your diet?

   a) Very high (I eat a lot of high-fat dairy products, meat, bakery products and snack foods)

   b) Moderately high (I use some lower-fat dairy products and lean red meat, and try to limit the amount of bakery products and snack foods)

    c) Very low (I eat a wide variety of grain products, vegetables and fruit and choose lower fat dairy products and lean meats)

5. If you take oral contraceptives, do you also smoke?

    a) Yes   b) No   c) Not applicable

What's Your Heart and Stroke I.Q.?

1. The signs and symptoms of coronary heart disease are:

    a) The same in both sexes

    b) Can be different in men and women

2. High blood pressure—hypertension—is caused by:

    a) Being tense and stressed

    b) Too much salt in the diet

    c) In most cases, we don't know what causes it

3. The following symptoms may occur alone or in combination:

- Sudden weakness or numbness of the face, arm or leg on one side
- Sudden dimness or loss of vision, particularly in one eye
- Sudden loss of speech, trouble talking or understanding speech
- Sudden severe headache with no apparent cause
- Unexplained dizziness, unsteadiness or sudden falls, especially along with any of the previous symptoms

These are symptoms of:

    a) Stroke   b) Angina Pectoris   c) Heart Attack

4. When you compare men and women who have heart attacks:

    a) Men are at greater risk of dying from a heart attack

    b) Women are at greater risk of dying from a heart attack

    c) Men and women are at equal risk of dying from a heart attack

5. After menopause, a woman's risk of heart disease and stroke:

   a) Decreases   b) Stays the same   c) Increases

Are You Ready to Take Charge?

1. What would you do if you experienced the following:

   - Pain, a feeling of tightness, pressure, or burning sensation in the chest and/or radiating down the arm or up into the neck or jaw
   - Difficulty breathing, shortness of breath, nausea or feeling of indigestion
   - A feeling of anxiety, sweating, weakness

     a) Go to bed and hope it goes away?

     b) Call 911 or emergency services?

2. How often do you have your blood pressure checked?

   a) Once every two years—more frequently, if your physician advises

   b) Once every five years

   c) Never

3. How often should your cholesterol level be checked?

   a) Never—only men need to have their cholesterol levels checked

   b) There is no one answer—it depends upon your age, risk factors for heart disease and stroke, and other health conditions

4. If your doctor prescribes medication to lower your blood pressure, you can safely skip taking it when:

   a) You're on vacation and feeling relaxed

   b) You run out and can't get to the store for a couple of days

   c) You can never skip your medication

5. The single best way of improving your diet would be to:

   a) Buy packaged foods that are labeled "cholesterol-free"

b) Increase the amount of fiber and decrease the amount of fat in your diet

c) Switch to sugar-free foods

6. Have you talked to your doctor about:

a) Smoking: how and when to quit

b) Approaching menopause: the benefits and risks of hormone replacement therapy

c) Family history of premature heart disease or stroke in your family: how to reduce your risk

d) None of the above

How Do You Rate?

Take a look and see where you need to do some work to improve your odds against the #1 killer of women.

Personal Risk Profile

_____/12 points
The higher your score, the greater your risk of heart disease and stroke. Talk to your doctor about your risk factors—and how you can control them.

Your Lifestyle Risk Profile

_____/14 points
The higher your score, the greater the risk your lifestyle is putting you for heart disease or stroke. Take charge now!

Your Heart And Stroke I.Q.

_____/10 points
The lower your score, the less you know about the #1 killer of Canadian women—heart disease and stroke.

Ready to Take Charge

_____/12 points
The lower your score, the less ready you are to take charge of your heart health. Learn to take charge.

Personal Risk Profile

Question/Answers/Your Score
1 a=2 points; b=0 points **2** a=2 points; b=0 points **3** a=2 points; b=0 points **4** a=2 points; b=0 points **5** a=2 points; b=0 points **6** a=2 points; b=1 points; c=0 points
Total:

Your Lifestyle Risk Profile

Question/Answers/Your Score
1 a=4 points; b=3 points; c=1 point; d=0 points **2** a=2 points; b=1 points **3** a=2 points; b=0 points **4** a=2 points; b=1 point; c=0 points **5** a=2 points; b=0 points; c=0 points
Total:

Your Heart and Stroke I.Q.

Question/Answers/Your Score
1 a=0 points; b=2 points **2** a=0 points; b=1 point; c=2 points **3** a=2 points; b=0 points; c=0 points **4** a=0 points; b=2 points; c=0 points **5** a=0 points; b=0 points; c=2 points
Total:

Ready to Take Charge

Question/Answers/Your Score
1 a=0 points; b=2 points **2** a=2 points; b=0 points; c=0 points **3** a=0 points; b=2 points **4** a=0 points; b=0 points; c=2 points **5** a=0 points; b=2 points; c=0 points **6** a=2 points; b=2 points; c=2 points; d=0 points
Total:

Chapter 6

The Heart

The heart is a muscular structure about the size of your fist, connected to the rest of your body by a 60,000-mile network of blood vessels. Shaped more like a cone than the Valentine we picture, the heart lies slightly to the left of the center of your chest, protected by the breastbone (sternum) in front, the spinal column in back, and the lungs and ribs on both sides. The heart is positioned so that the tip of the cone points toward your left hip.

In a lifetime, the human heart will typically beat 2.5 billion times. That amounts to about once a second, every minute of your life—considerably faster during exercise and slower when you sleep. Although the heart only weighs between 7 and 15 ounces (depending on your size and weight), it can pump five or more quarts of blood a minute. Each day, your heart pumps about 2,000 gallons of blood throughout your body—enough blood in a lifetime to fill more than three supertankers—and is strong enough to drive a single drop of blood throughout your entire body in about 24 seconds.

The heart's pumping action consists of squeezing blood out of its chambers (contracting), and then expanding to allow blood to flow back in (relaxation). The action is as simple as squeezing water out of a soft plastic bottle while holding it under water and then releasing your grasp so water is sucked back into the bottle as it expands.

Johns Hopkins InteliHealth (www.intelihealth.com), © 1997 The Johns Hopkins University; reprinted with permission of InteliHealth. Illustrations are from "The Human Heart: A Living Pump," National Heart, Lung, and Blood Institute, NIH Pub. No. 95-1059.

This cycle of contraction and relaxation, the heartbeat, creates the pulse you can feel in your wrist. Doctors look at two measures to determine the strength of the heart muscle: ejection fraction and cardiac output.

Ejection fraction: No matter how forceful your heart's contraction, it doesn't pump all the blood out of the ventricles with each beat. The portion of blood pumped out of a filled ventricle is referred to as the ejection fraction. A normal ejection fraction of about 60 to 65 percent means that about two-thirds of the blood in the ventricles is pumped out with each beat. The ejection fraction is a good indicator of the overall function of the heart. In a healthy person, the ejection fraction increases about 5 percent with exercise. However, when the ventricles are diseased, as a result of a heart attack or other heart disorders, the ejection fraction can fall to 30 percent.

Cardiac output: The actual amount of blood pumped by the left ventricle during one contraction is called the stroke volume. The stroke volume and the heart rate determine the cardiac output, which is the amount of blood the heart pumps through the entire circulatory system in one minute.

Parts of the heart include:

- Chambers
- Protective Membranes
- Valves
- The Conduction System
- The Cardiac Cycle

Chambers

The heart is divided into four chambers—the right atrium, the left atrium, the right ventricle and the left ventricle. The upper chambers (the atria) receive blood, while the lower chambers (ventricles) pump blood. The left and right atria and the left and right ventricles are separated from each other by a wall of muscle called the septum.

Blood returning from the rest of the body enters the heart through the right atrium, which acts as something of a storage bin. After collecting in the right atrium, blood enters the right ventricle. As the right ventricle contracts, it pumps the blood into the lungs, where it is enriched with oxygen. Pulmonary veins in the lungs then bring the oxygen-enriched blood to the left atrium, where it collects until it is pushed into the left ventricle, the main pumping chamber of the heart. The left ventricle pumps the blood through the aorta and into the circulatory system, where it is distributed to the entire body.

In a healthy heart, blood cannot flow between the right and left sides. The atria are separated by a wall called the atrial septum, and the ventricles by the ventricular septum.

Protective Membranes

The outside surface of the heart is covered by a thin, glossy membrane called the epicardium. Another smooth, glossy membrane, the endocardium, covers the inside surfaces of the four heart chambers,

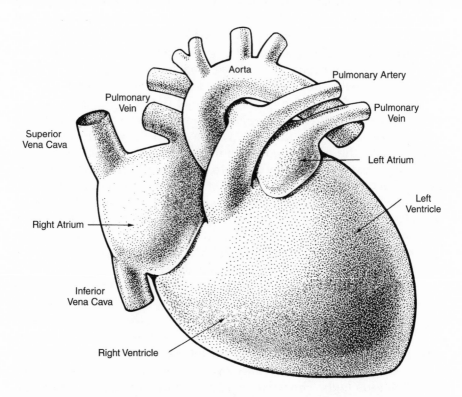

Figure 6.1. *The heart is a hollow, muscular organ with four chambers. The upper two are blood-receiving chambers called atria. The lower two are blood-pumping chambers called ventricles.*

plus the valves and the muscles that attach to the valves. The entire heart is enveloped in two sacs called the pericardium. A small amount of fluid between the two sacs acts as a lubricant, allowing the heart to beat with minimal friction. The inner sac of the pericardium is a thin, moist membrane, which cushions the heart. The tough outer layer attaches to several areas in the chest to anchor the heart in place. When the heart muscle contracts, the pumping chambers become smaller, squeezing blood out of the heart. When the heart muscle relaxes, the pumping chambers expand and blood flows back into the heart.

Valves

Although the pumping action of your heart is certainly effective at ejecting blood from its chambers, it also needs a method to guarantee that the pumped blood goes only in the desired direction. This task falls to four heart valves: the tricuspid, mitral, pulmonary, and aortic. The valves are strong, thin leaflets of tissue anchored to the myocardium. The flaps consist of single sheets of fibrous tissue covered by endocardial cells. At the base of each valve leaflet, the fibrous layer merges with the myocardium to form a flexible hinge.

The tricuspid valve (on the right side of the heart) and the mitral valve (on the left side) regulate blood flow from the atria to the ventricles. The aortic and pulmonary valves guard the openings from the ventricles to the aortic and pulmonary arteries, respectively. The valves are designed to allow blood to pass in only one direction. The valves don't automatically open when blood is approaching. Instead, they function like a gate that opens only when it's pushed and is designed so that it can swing open in only one direction. The valves open and close due to the natural pressure differences that build up within the heart's chambers during the systolic and diastolic portions of each cardiac cycle [*see* "The Cardiac Cycle" below].

For example, the aortic valve opens to allow blood to eject from the left ventricle into the aorta, because during systole (contraction) the pressure in the left ventricle is higher than in the aorta. This pressure difference forces the valve to open and allows blood to flow through it. During diastole, when the left ventricle relaxes, the pressure in the left ventricle becomes low again while the pressure in the aorta remains high. The valve is pushed closed by the pressure, and blood is prevented from leaking back into the heart.

The familiar sound of the heartbeat is caused by the heart valves slamming shut. The first thump is heard when the valves between the atria and ventricles close; the second when the valves between the ventricles and arteries close.

The Conduction System

The intricate timing system that controls the rhythmic beating of your heart is handled by the heart's electrical, or conduction system. This system is the circuitry that conducts electrical impulses throughout the muscle of the heart. These electrical impulses stimulate the heart muscle to contract and squeeze blood out of the heart and into the arteries.

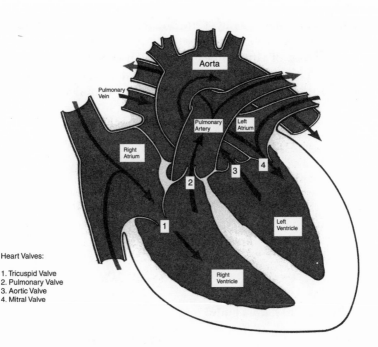

Figure 6.2. Oxygen-poor blood from the body flows down through the right atrium to fill the right ventricle which pumps the blood out through the pulmonary artery to the lungs. Oxygen-rich blood from the lungs flows down through the left atrium to fill the left ventricle which pumps it into the aorta, the main artery to the body. The four heart valves: the tricuspid, mitral, pulmonary, and aortic, regulate the direction of blood flow.

41

The sinus node, the heart's natural pacemaker, consists of a group of cells in the upper part of the right atrium. Also called the sinoatrial node, it's the normal point of origin of the electrical impulses.

Once the electrical signal is generated by the sinus node, it moves from cell to cell down through the heart until it reaches the atrioventricular (AV) node, a cluster of cells in the center of the heart between the atria and ventricles. The AV node acts as a gate that slows the electrical current before it's allowed to pass through to the ventricles. This delay ensures that the atria have had a chance to fully contract before the ventricles are stimulated.

After clearing the AV node, the electrical current is channeled to the ventricles by special fibers embedded in the walls of the lower parts of the heart. It's this transfer of electrical impulses that doctors measure when they take an electrocardiogram to measure how well a heart is beating.

The autonomic nervous system, the same system that automatically controls blood pressure, breathing and excretion, for example, controls the firing of the sinus node, which triggers the start of the cardiac cycle. This system can make snap decisions, causing the sinus node to increase the heart rate to twice normal within only 3 to

Table 6.1. Heart Rates for Different Ages

Normal Heart Rates at Rest

Age Group	Beats per Minute
Newborn	140
Young Child	100-120
Adult	60-100

Maximal Attainable Heart Rates

Age in Years	Beats per Minute
25	200
35	188
45	176
55	165
65	155

5 seconds. This flexibility is important during exercise, when the heart must rapidly increase its beating speed to keep up with the body's increased demand for oxygen.

As you age, your heart rate slows. The decrease is not noticeable during everyday activities, but your maximal heart rate during exercise decreases as you grow older. For example, your maximal heart rate at age 25 is about 200 beats per minute; by age 65, it has dropped to about 155 beats per minute.

The Cardiac Cycle

The pathway of the electrical impulses can best be seen by looking in detail at a single heart cycle. The period from the beginning of one heartbeat to the next is called the cardiac cycle. The cardiac cycle consists of a period of contraction, called systole, followed by a period of relaxation, called diastole. During the diastole phase, your heart relaxes and allows blood to flow into the two ventricles; during the systole phase, the ventricles contract, driving blood to the lungs and throughout the body. In a healthy, resting adult, the heart beats about 70 to 75 times a minute, so that the cardiac cycle lasts only about .8 seconds.

Part Two

Major Risk Factors
and Prevention

Chapter 7

Major Risk Factors in Women

Smoking

Cigarette smoking has been described as "the most important individual health risk in this country." Approximately 23 million American women smoke. Although the smoking rate for women dropped 11 percent between 1965 and 1990, women who smoke today are apt to smoke more heavily than they did in the past.

Surprising as it may seem, smoking by women in the United States causes almost as many deaths from heart disease as from lung cancer. Women who smoke are two to six times as likely to suffer a heart attack as nonsmoking women, and the risk increases with the number of cigarettes smoked per day. Smoking also boosts the risk of stroke.

Cardiovascular diseases are not the only health risks for women who smoke. Cigarette smoking greatly increases the chances that a woman will develop lung cancer. In fact, the lung cancer death rate for women is now higher than the death rate for breast cancer, the chief cause of cancer deaths in women for many years. Cigarette smoking is also linked with cancers of the mouth, larynx, esophagus, urinary tract, kidney, pancreas, and cervix. Smoking also causes 80 percent of cases of chronic obstructive lung disease, which includes bronchitis and emphysema.

Excerpted from *Heart Healthy Handbook for Women,* National Heart, Lung, and Blood Institute (NHLBI), NIH Publication No. 97-2720, revised July 1997.

Smoking is also linked to a number of reproductive problems. Women who smoke are more apt to have problems getting pregnant and to begin menopause at a slightly younger age. Further, cigarette use during pregnancy poses serious risks for the unborn. Babies of women who smoked during pregnancy tend to weigh less at birth than babies of nonsmokers. Smoking while pregnant also increases risks of bleeding, miscarriage, premature delivery, stillbirth, and sudden infant death syndrome, or "crib death." Moreover, young children who are exposed to a parent's cigarette smoke have more lung and ear infections.

There is simply no safe way to smoke. Although low-tar and low nicotine cigarettes may reduce the lung cancer risk to some extent, they do not lessen the risks of heart disease or other smoking-related diseases. The only safe and healthful course is not to smoke at all.

High Blood Pressure

High blood pressure, also known as hypertension, is another major risk factor for coronary heart disease and the most important risk factor for stroke. Even slightly high levels double the risk. High blood pressure also increases the chances of developing congestive heart failure and kidney disease.

Nearly 50 million Americans have high blood pressure, and about half of them are women. Older women have a higher risk, with more than half of all women over the age of 55 suffering from this condition. High blood pressure is more common and more severe in African-American women than it is in white women. Use of birth control pills can contribute to high blood pressure in some women.

Blood pressure is the amount of force exerted by the blood against the walls of the arteries. Everyone has to have some blood pressure, so that blood can get to the body's organs and muscles. Usually, blood pressure is expressed as two numbers, such as 120/80, and is measured in millimeters of mercury (mmHg). The first number is the systolic blood pressure, the force used when the heart beats. The second number, or diastolic blood pressure, is the pressure that exists in the arteries between heartbeats. Depending on your activities, blood pressure may move up or down in the course of a day. Blood pressure is considered high when it stays above normal levels over a period of time.

High blood pressure is sometimes called the "silent killer" because most people who have it do not feel sick. Therefore, it is important to have it checked whenever you see your doctor or other health professional. Blood pressure can be easily measured by means of the familiar stethoscope and inflatable cuff placed around one arm. However, since blood pressure changes so often and is affected by many factors, your health professional should check it on several different days before deciding whether your blood pressure is too high. If your blood pressure stays at 140/90 mmHg or above, you have high blood pressure.

Although high blood pressure can rarely be cured, it can be controlled with proper treatment. If your blood pressure is not too high, you may be able to control it entirely through weight loss if you are overweight, regular physical activity, and cutting down on alcohol, and salt and sodium. (Sodium is an ingredient in salt that is found in many packaged foods, carbonated beverages, baking soda, and some antacids.)

It may also help to include more fruits and vegetables that are good sources of potassium, and low and nonfat dairy products and some vegetables that are good sources of calcium.

However, if your blood pressure remains high, your doctor will probably prescribe medicine in addition to the above changes, especially if you already have heart disease. The lifestyle changes described above will help the medicine work more effectively. In fact, if you are successful with the changes you make in your living habits, the amount of medicine you take may be gradually reduced.

While few people like the idea of taking any medicine for a long time, the treatment benefits are real and will reduce the risk of stroke, heart attack, congestive heart failure, and kidney disease. If you are prescribed a drug to control high blood pressure and have any uncomfortable side effects, ask your doctor about changing the dosage or possibly switching to another type of medicine.

A *reminder*: It is very important to take a blood pressure medication exactly as your doctor has prescribed it. If you are not sure about your doctor's instructions, call to ask about the amount of medicine you are supposed to take each day, and the specific times of day you should be taking it.

During pregnancy, some women develop high blood pressure for the first time. Between 10 and 20 percent of first-time mothers develop a high blood pressure problem during pregnancy called preeclampsia. Other women who already have high blood pressure may find that it worsens during pregnancy. If untreated, these conditions can be life threatening to both mother and baby. Since a woman can feel perfectly normal and still have one of these conditions, it is important to get regular prenatal checkups so that your doctor can discover and treat a possible high blood pressure problem.

For women with a type of high blood pressure called isolated systolic hypertension (ISH), there is good news. By treating ISH with a blood pressure-lowering drug such as a diuretic, it is possible to reduce the risk of stroke and coronary heart disease. If you know you have ISH and are already doing well on another type of blood pressure-lowering drug, you should not necessarily switch medicines. But you may want to discuss with your doctor whether or not you have ISH and, if so, what is the best treatment for you.

High Blood Cholesterol

High blood cholesterol is another important risk factor for coronary heart disease that you can do something about. All women should keep their cholesterol levels down to lessen the chance of developing heart disease. For those who already have heart disease, it is particularly important to take action to treat elevated blood cholesterol to prevent a future heart attack.

Although young women tend to have lower cholesterol levels than young men, between the ages of 45 and 55, women's cholesterol levels begin to rise higher than men's. After age 55, the gap between women and men becomes still wider. The higher a woman's blood cholesterol level, the higher her heart disease risk. Today, about one-quarter of American women have blood cholesterol levels high enough to pose a serious risk for coronary heart disease.

Cholesterol and the Heart

The body needs cholesterol to function normally. However, the body makes all of the cholesterol that it needs. Over a period of years, extra cholesterol and fat circulating in the blood are deposited in the walls of the arteries that supply blood to the heart. These deposits make the arteries narrower and narrower. As a result, less blood gets to the heart and the risk of coronary heart disease increases.

Cholesterol travels in the blood in packages called lipoproteins. Low density lipoprotein (LDL) carries most of the cholesterol in the blood. Cholesterol packaged in LDL is often called "bad" cholesterol, because too much LDL in blood can lead to cholesterol buildup and blockage in the arteries.

Another type of cholesterol, which is packaged in high density lipoprotein (HDL), is known as "good cholesterol." That is because HDL helps remove cholesterol from the blood, preventing it from piling up in the arteries.

50

All women over the age of 20 should have their blood cholesterol checked. However, the testing process and the steps to improve cholesterol levels will depend on your current health status. The following sections describe the steps for managing cholesterol levels for two types of women: those who do not have heart disease, and those who do have heart disease.

If You Do Not Have Heart Disease

Getting Your Cholesterol Checked. Blood cholesterol levels are measured by means of a small blood sample. The blood should be tested for total cholesterol and, if an accurate measurement is available, for HDL cholesterol as well. You do not have to fast or do anything special before having this blood test.

Understanding the Numbers. A desirable total cholesterol level for adults without heart disease is less than 200 mg/dL (or 200 milligrams of cholesterol per deciliter of blood). A level of 240 mg/dL or above is considered "high" blood cholesterol. But even levels in the "borderline-high" category (200-239 mg/dL) still increase the risk of heart disease.

Before age 45, the total blood cholesterol level of women averages below 200 mg/dL. But between the ages of 45 and 55, women's average cholesterol level rises to almost 220 mg/dL, and to nearly 240 mg/dL for women between the ages of 55 and 64. Women who have a cholesterol level over 240 mg/dL are more than twice as likely to develop heart disease as women with levels below 200 mg/dL.

HDL levels are interpreted differently than total cholesterol levels. The lower your HDL level, the higher your heart disease risk. An HDL level of under 35 is a major risk factor for heart disease. The higher your level, the less risk you incur. A level of 60 or higher is considered protective.

Total and HDL-cholesterol are measured first. Depending on what these initial measurements show and whether you have any other heart disease risk factors, your doctor may want to measure your LDL level as well. For this test, you should have nothing to eat or drink except water (or black coffee or tea) for 9-12 hours beforehand.

An LDL level below 130 mg/dL is desirable. LDL levels of 130-159 mg/dL are borderline-high. Levels of 160 mg/dL or above are high. As with total cholesterol, the higher the LDL number, the higher the risk.

Prevention and Treatment. If your tests show that your blood cholesterol levels are in the desirable range, congratulations! To help keep your levels healthy, it will be important to eat a low saturated fat, low cholesterol diet, get regular physical activity, and control your weight. Saturated fat raises your blood cholesterol more than anything else in your diet.

If your blood cholesterol levels are too high, your doctor may recommend a specific treatment program for you. For most people, cutting back on foods high in saturated fat and cholesterol will lower both total and LDL-cholesterol. Regular physical activity and weight loss for overweight persons also will lower blood cholesterol levels.

Losing extra weight, as well as quitting smoking and becoming more physically active, also may help boost your HDL-cholesterol levels. Although we don't know for sure that raising HDL levels in this way will reduce the risk of coronary heart disease, these measures are likely to be good for your heart in any case.

If your new diet and other lifestyle changes do not lower your blood cholesterol level enough, your doctor may suggest that you take cholesterol-lowering medications. If you have other risk factors for heart disease, you will need to lower your cholesterol more than someone without risk factors.

If You Have Heart Disease

Women who have heart disease should pay even more attention to their cholesterol levels. An individual with heart disease has a much greater risk of having a future heart attack than a person without heart disease. Recent studies show that, even if your cholesterol level is not elevated, lowering it can greatly reduce your risk of a future heart attack and may actually prolong your life.

Getting Your Cholesterol Checked. Since you have heart disease, you will need to have a blood test called a lipoprotein profile. This test will determine not only your total cholesterol and HDL-cholesterol levels, but also your LDL-cholesterol level and levels of another fatty substance called triglycerides. In order to take this test, you should have nothing to eat or drink except water (or coffee or tea with no cream or sugar) for 9-12 hours beforehand.

Understanding the Numbers. Your goal should be to have an LDL-cholesterol level of about 100 mg/dL or less, which is lower than for people who do not have heart disease. Depending on what your LDL level is, your next steps will be the following:

- *If your LDL level is 100 mg/dL or less,* you do not need to take specific steps to lower your LDL. But you will need to have your level tested again in 1 year. In the meantime, you should closely follow a diet low in saturated fat and cholesterol, maintain a healthy weight, be physically active, and not smoke. You should also follow the specific recommendations of your doctor.

- *If your LDL level is higher than 100 mg/dL,* you will need a complete physical examination to find out if you have a disease or condition that is raising your cholesterol levels. You will probably need a diet that is very low in saturated fat and cholesterol. In addition, you will need to be physically active, lose weight if you are overweight, and not smoke.

If in your doctor's judgment, your LDL level starts out too far above the LDL goal of 100 mg/dL or if your LDL level stays too high after lifestyle changes, you may need to take medicine. For many individuals, it is necessary to combine medication with lifestyle changes to get enough of a reduction in LDL-cholesterol. Your doctor can help to decide which combination of cholesterol-lowering activities is right for you.

Overweight

Overweight women are much more likely to develop heart-related problems even if they have no other risk factors. According to a long-term study of nearly 116,000 women, almost 40 percent of coronary heart disease was attributed to overweight. For the heaviest women, 72 percent of coronary heart disease could be traced to excess weight. The study also showed that even a modest weight gain of 11-17 pounds after age 18 significantly increases a woman's risk of coronary heart disease.

Overweight also appears to contribute to cardiovascular disease in part by increasing the chance of developing other risk factors, such as high blood pressure, high blood cholesterol, and diabetes. However, it also appears that obesity is harmful even in the absence of these conditions. Fortunately, these conditions often can be controlled by maintaining a healthy weight and by getting regular physical activity.

What is a healthy weight for you? Currently, there is no exact answer. Researchers are trying to develop better ways to measure healthy weight.

Those who are currently overweight should take special care not to gain additional pounds, since the more overweight a person is, the higher the chances of developing heart disease. Research also suggests that body shape as well as weight affects heart health. "Apple-shaped" individuals with extra fat at the waistline may have a higher risk than "pear-shaped" people with heavy hips and thighs. If your waist is as large as the size of your hips, or larger, you may have a higher risk for coronary heart disease.

Physical Inactivity

Physical inactivity increases the risk of heart disease. It both contributes directly to heart-related problems and increases the chances of developing other risk factors, such as high blood pressure and diabetes.

Recent reports from the U.S. Surgeon General's Office and a National Institutes of Health (NIH) expert panel warn that physical inactivity is increasing among Americans—especially among women.

According to the first-ever Surgeon General's Report on Physical Activity and Health, 60 percent of American women don't get the recommended amount of physical activity, while more than 25 percent are not active at all. In part, this sedentary behavior results from a reliance on modern conveniences, such as automobiles, elevators, and escalators, which make life easier but do little to strengthen or tone the body, but even during leisure hours, many women continue to be physically inactive.

This inactivity can have serious results later in life. Besides increasing the risk of heart disease, it makes older woman who are not physically active more likely to fall than those who are physically active. And, especially for those with bone loss, falls can lead to fractures and have serious, even life-threatening, consequences.

Fortunately, it doesn't take a lot of effort to become physically active. Both the Surgeon General's report and the report of the NIH Consensus Development Conference on Physical Activity and Cardiovascular Health conclude that as little as 30 minutes of moderate activity on most, and preferably all, days helps protect heart health. Examples of moderate activity are a brisk walk, raking leaves, or gardening.

If you prefer, you can divide the 30-minute activity into shorter periods of at least 10 minutes each. If you already do this level of activity, you can get added benefits by doing even more.

Diabetes

Diabetes is a serious disorder that raises the risk of coronary heart disease and stroke. About 75 percent of people who have diabetes die of some type of cardiovascular disease.

Compared with nondiabetic women, diabetic women are more apt to have high blood pressure and high blood cholesterol. Untreated diabetes also can contribute to the development of kidney disease, blindness, problems in pregnancy and childbirth, nerve and blood vessel damage, and difficulties in fighting infection.

The type of diabetes that develops in adulthood is usually "noninsulin-dependent diabetes mellitus," or NIDDM. This type of diabetes, in which the pancreas makes insulin but the body is unable to use it well, is the most common form of the disease. For unknown reasons, the risks of heart disease and heart-related death are higher for diabetic women than for diabetic men.

While there is no cure for diabetes, there are steps one can take to control it. About 80 percent of all NIDDM diabetics are overweight. It appears that overweight and growing older promote the development of diabetes in certain people. Losing weight and increasing physical activity may help postpone or prevent the disease. For lasting weight loss, engage in regular, brisk physical activity and eat a diet that is limited in calories and fat.

Other Factors

Stress

In recent years, we have read and heard much about the connection between stress and coronary heart disease. And many studies do report such a connection for both women and men. For example, the most commonly reported incident preceding a heart attack is an emotionally upsetting event, particularly one that involves anger. There also is evidence that people who become easily emotionally upset are more likely to develop hardening of the arteries. In addition, some common ways of coping with stress, such as overeating, heavy drinking, and smoking, are clearly bad for your heart.

The good news is that sensible health habits can have a protective effect. Regular physical activity not only relieves stress, but can directly lower your risk of heart disease. Recent research also shows that involvement in a stress management program following a heart attack decreases the chances of further heart-related problems.

Strong personal ties may also play an important role in heart disease management and prevention. Studies show that having emotionally supportive relationships lessens the chances of developing heart disease, and prolongs life in both women and men following a heart attack. Religious beliefs and activity also have been linked to longer survival among heart surgery patients. While these findings are promising, researchers will need to study larger groups of women over time to find out more about the links among certain behaviors, stress, and coronary heart disease in women.

Birth Control Pills

Studies show that women who use high-dose birth control pills (oral contraceptives) are more likely to have a heart attack or a stroke because blood clots are more likely to form in the blood vessels. These risks are lessened once the birth control pill is stopped. Using birth control pills also may worsen the effects of other risk factors, such as smoking, high blood pressure, diabetes, high blood cholesterol, and overweight.

Much of this information comes from studies of birth control pills containing higher doses of hormones than those commonly used today. Still, the risks of using low-dose birth control pills are not fully known. Therefore, if you are now taking any kind of birth control pill or are considering using one, keep these guidelines in mind:

- *Smoking and "the pill" don't mix.* If you smoke cigarettes, stop smoking or choose a different form of birth control. Cigarette smoking boosts the risk of serious cardiovascular problems from birth control pill use, especially the risk of blood clots. This risk increases with age and with the amount smoked. For women over 35, the risk is particularly high. Women who use oral contraceptives should not smoke.

- *Pay attention to diabetes.* Glucose metabolism, or blood sugar, sometimes changes dramatically in women who take birth control pills. Any woman who is diabetic, or has a close relative who is, should have regular blood sugar tests if she takes birth control pills.

- *Watch your blood pressure.* After starting to take birth control pills, your blood pressure may go up. For most women, this increase does not go above normal. But if your blood pressure increases to 140/90 mmHg or higher, ask your doctor about changing pills or switching to another form of birth control. Once off birth control pills, your blood pressure should return to normal within a few months.

- *Talk with your doctor.* If you have a heart defect, if you have suffered a stroke, or if you have any other kind of cardiovascular disease, oral contraceptives may not be a safe choice. Be sure your doctor knows about your condition before prescribing birth control pills for you.

Alcohol

Over the last several years, a number of studies have reported that moderate drinkers—those who have one or two drinks per day—are less likely to develop heart disease than people who don't drink any alcohol or who drink too much. Small amounts of alcohol may help protect against heart disease by raising levels of "good" HDL cholesterol.

If you are a nondrinker, this is not a recommendation to start using alcohol. And certainly if you are pregnant, planning to become pregnant, or have another health condition that could make alcohol use harmful, you should not drink. But if you're already a moderate drinker, evidence suggests that you may be at a lower risk for heart attack. This is particularly true for women after menopause.

But remember, moderation is the key. Heavy drinking causes heart related problems. More than three drinks per day can raise blood pressure, and binge drinking can contribute to stroke. Too much alcohol also may damage the heart muscle, leading to heart failure. Overall, people who drink heavily on a regular basis have higher rates of heart disease than either moderate drinkers or nondrinkers.

Women who drink should have no more than one alcoholic beverage a day.

Keep in mind, too, that alcohol provides no nutrients—only extra calories. Most alcoholic drinks contain 100-200 calories each. Women who are trying to control their weight may want to cut down on alcohol and substitute calorie-free iced tea, mineral water, or seltzer with a squeeze of lemon or lime.

What Is Moderate Drinking?

For women, moderate drinking is defined as no more than one drink per day, according to the U.S. Dietary Guidelines for Americans. Count as one drink:

- 12 ounces of regular beer (150 calories)
- 5 ounces of wine (100 calories)
- 1 1/2 ounces of 80-proof hard liquor (100 calories)

Source: *Dietary Guidelines for Americans,* U.S. Department of Agriculture/U.S. Department of Health and Human Services, 1995.

Homocysteine

Homocysteine (pronounced homo-SIS-teen) is an amino acid found normally in the body. Recent studies suggest that high levels of this substance may increase a person's chances of developing heart disease, stroke, and reduced blood flow to the hands and feet. While it is not known for sure how homocysteine contributes to heart and vessel disease, it is thought that high levels of homocysteine may damage the arteries, make the blood more likely to clot, and/or make blood vessels less flexible.

Individuals vary in their levels of homocysteine. For a few people, genetic factors contribute to high amounts of this substance in the blood. In addition, homocysteine levels may increase with age. For women, homocysteine levels may be higher after menopause than during childbearing years.

Recent research also shows that the level of homocysteine in the blood is affected by the consumption of three vitamins—folic acid, and vitamins B6 and B12. People who consume less than the recommended daily amounts of these vitamins are more likely to have higher homocysteine levels. Recommended daily amounts are as follows:

- 400 micrograms for folic acid
- 2 milligrams for B6
- 6 micrograms for B12

It has not yet been proven that lowering homocysteine levels will actually help to prevent heart or blood vessel disease. But until more research is done, people may help protect their health by getting enough folic acid, B6, and B 12 in their diets.

Good sources of folic acid include citrus fruits, tomatoes, vegetables, whole- and fortified-grain products, beans and lentils. Beginning in 1998, the U.S. Food and Drug Administration will require that certain foods contain extra folic acid to help prevent certain birth defects. These foods include enriched breads and rolls, all enriched flours, corn meals, all enriched pasta products, and breakfast cereals.

Foods high in B6 include meat, poultry, fish, fruits, vegetables and grain products. Major sources of B12 are meat, poultry, fish, and milk and other dairy products.

Are Calcium Channel Blockers Safe?

A few people with high blood pressure certain heart disorders take a medication known as short-acting or nifedipine, which is a type of calcium channel blocker (CCB). Recent research, however, found that patients taking short-acting nifedipine—especially in high doses—were more likely to have another heart attack, and also more likely to die of a heart attack. As a result, physicians have been advised to prescribe this particular medication to patients with caution, if at all, or to change to another kind of medication.

It is important to understand, however, that short-acting nifedipine is one of several kinds of CCBs. It is unclear whether the other types, such as verapamil and diltiazem, are also risky. Also, some CCBs are available in two forms, short-acting (requiring several daily doses) and long-acting (requiring one daily dose). While short-acting nifedipine does increase heart attack risk, it is not yet known whether the long-acting form of nifedipine also increases risk.

If you are currently taking short-acting nifedipine, talk with your doctor as soon as possible to find out whether you should switch to another medication. If you are taking another kind of CCB, you might also want to ask your doctor about other medication choices.

This new information should not discourage you from taking medicine for high blood pressure or heart disorders. Drug treatment for high blood pressure helps prevent stroke, heart attack, congestive heart failure, and kidney disease. Other types of medication, such as diuretics and beta-blockers, are safe and effective treatments for most people with high blood pressure.

Congestive Heart Failure: Another Reason to Control Your Blood Pressure

High blood pressure is the number one risk factor for congestive heart failure (CHF). Heart failure is a serious condition in which the heart is unable to pump enough blood to supply the body's needs. As a result, blood gets backed up in the veins and begins to seep into surrounding tissues. CHF occurs when excess fluid starts to leak into the lungs, causing breathing difficulties, fatigue and weakness, and sleeping problems.

In recent years, rates of hospitalization and death for CHF have been increasing in older Americans, especially among women. One reason may be that many women do not adequately control their high blood pressure. Older women must be especially careful to continue taking blood pressure medication regularly—and also to take the right amount. To prevent CHF, and stroke as well, blood pressure must be controlled to 140/90 mmHg or lower. However, many women who are taking medication still have blood pressure that is dangerously high. If your blood pressure is higher than 140/90 mmHg, talk with your doctor about adjusting your medication and making lifestyle changes that will result in a blood pressure of 140/90 mmHg or lower.

Next Steps

If your total cholesterol is less than 200 mg/dL and HDL is 35 mg/dL or greater, then you are doing well and should have your total and HDL-cholesterol levels checked again in about 5 years. In the meantime, take steps to keep your total-cholesterol level down by eating foods low in saturated fat and cholesterol, maintaining a healthy weight, and being physically active. The last two steps, along with not smoking, will also help keep your HDL level up.

If your total cholesterol is 200-239 mg/dL and HDL is 35 mg/dL or greater, then your doctor will see if you have other risk factors for heart disease and determine whether more tests (including a lipoprotein profile to find out your LDL-cholesterol) need to be done. No matter what your risk is, it is important to eat foods low in saturated fat and cholesterol, to maintain a healthy weight, and to be physically active.

If your total cholesterol is 240 mg/dL or greater or HDL is less than 35 mg/dL, then you will need a lipoprotein profile to find out your LDL-cholesterol level. You need to fast for 9-12 hours before the test, having nothing but water, or coffee or tea with no cream or sugar.

What's Your Number?

Table 7.1. Blood Cholesterol Levels and Heart Disease Risk*

	Desirable	Borderline-High	High
Total Cholesterol	Less than 200	200-239	240 and above
LDL Cholesterol	Less than 130	130-159	160 and above

HDL-cholesterol less than 35 is a major risk factor for heart disease. HDL 60 or higher is protective.

*For women without heart disease.

60

Cholesterol-Lowering Medicines

Your doctor may recommend medication as part of your cholesterol-lowering treatment plan. This is more likely if you have heart disease, if you have very high LDL levels, or if you have high blood cholesterol in combination with other heart disease risk factors.

If your doctor does prescribe medicines, you must also continue your cholesterol-lowering diet along with physical activity and weight control. These lifestyle changes lower your risk in many ways, not just by lowering your cholesterol levels, and the combination of lifestyle and medicine may allow you to take less medication. The most commonly used cholesterol-lowering medicines are as follows:

- *Hormone Replacement Therapy.* If you have reached menopause, your doctor may recommend that you begin hormone replacement therapy, which has many effects including raising HDL levels and lowering LDL levels.

- *Statins.* Statins are used by patients with high total and high LDL-cholesterol levels. Of all the available medications, statins lower LDL-cholesterol the most, producing reductions of 20-60 percent. Currently available statins are lovastatin, simvastatin, pravastatin, fluvastatin, and atorvastatin. Side effects are usually mild, although liver and muscle problems occur rarely.

- *Bile Acid Sequestrants.* The major effect of this medication is to lower LDL cholesterol by about 10 to 20 percent. Bile acid sequestrants are often prescribed with statin medicine for patients with heart disease to increase cholesterol reduction. Side effects may include constipation, bloating, nausea, and gas. However, long-term use of these medications is considered safe.

- *Nicotinic Acid.* Nicotinic acid, or niacin, lowers total cholesterol, LDL cholesterol, and triglyceride levels, while raising HDL-cholesterol levels. While nicotinic acid is available without a prescription, it is very important to use it only under a doctor's care, because of possibly serious side effects. In some people, nicotinic acid may inflame peptic ulcers or cause liver problems, gout, or high blood sugar.

What Are Triglycerides?

Triglycerides are another type of fat found in the blood and in food. Triglycerides are made up of saturated, polyunsaturated, and monounsaturated fats. They are produced in the liver. When alcohol or excess calories are taken in, the liver produces more triglycerides. Extremely high levels of triglycerides can cause a dangerous inflammation of the pancreas called pancreatitis. Fortunately, this is uncommon. Some people with coronary heart disease have high triglyceride levels. However, more research is needed to determine whether high triglycerides themselves cause narrowing of the arteries or are simply associated with other blood fat abnormalities and other risk factors (such as low levels of HDL-cholesterol and being overweight), which may increase the risk for coronary heart disease. Most people with raised triglycerides are also overweight, and weight reduction usually lowers the elevated levels.

To reduce blood triglyceride levels, doctors recommend a low fat, low-calorie diet, weight control, more physical activity, and no alcohol. Occasionally, medication is needed.

Chapter 8

Age at Menopause As a Risk Factor

Summary

Background. Although an association of occurrence of menopause and subsequent estrogen deficiency with increased cardiovascular disease has been postulated, studies on this association have not shown convincing results. We investigated whether age at menopause is associated with cardiovascular mortality risk.

Methods. We studied a cohort of 12,115 postmenopausal women living in Utrecht, Netherlands, aged 50-65 years at enrollment in a breast cancer screening project. During follow-up of up to 20 years the women attended screening rounds at which we asked questions on menopausal status, age at menopause, medication use, cardiovascular risk factors, and ovarian function. Deaths were ascertained from the patient's family physicians. Life-table analysis and Cox regression analysis were used to investigate the association between age at menopause and cardiovascular mortality. All analyses were adjusted for biological age.

Findings. 824 women died of cardiovascular causes. 1,459 women had left the study area. The risk of cardiovascular mortality was higher for women with early menopause than for those with late

The Lancet, March 16, 1996, Vol. 347, No. 9003, Pg. 714(5), by Yvonne T. van der Schouw, Yolanda van der Graaf, Ewout W. Steyerberg, Marinus J.C. Eijkemans, and Jan Dirk Banga, © 1996 Lancet Ltd.; reprinted with permission.

menopause. The extra risk of early menopause seemed to decrease with biological age. At biological age 60 the reduction of the annual hazard was 3%, but at age 80 there was no reduction. Adjustment for known cardiovascular risk factors and indicators of ovarian function did not significantly alter the risk estimate.

Interpretation. These results support the hypothesis that longer exposure to endogenous estrogens protects against cardiovascular diseases. The effect of an early menopause may be more important at younger biological ages.

Introduction

Premenopausal women seem to be protected against cardiovascular morbidity and mortality in comparison with men of similar age or postmenopausal women.[1-3] Loss of ovarian function and subsequent deficiency of endogenous estrogens is suggested to promote cardiovascular disease and death after menopause.[4,5]

If endogenous estrogens protect against cardiovascular disease, an early menopause might incur a higher risk, because of lower exposure to estrogens. Evidence for this hypothesis has been inconclusive.[6] Several investigations had small samples[5,7-9] and angina pectoris was used as the endpoint in some.[5,10,11] The two prospective studies that have been done, the Framingham Heart Study[2] and the Nurses' Health Study,[3] were better designed to address the question of whether the menopause itself is a risk factor for cardiovascular disease than to show whether an early menopause poses a particular risk. The main problem of studies done so far is the short postmenopausal follow-up period, which has probably been too short for cardiovascular diseases to occur in sufficient frequency for statistical analysis.

To explore the relation between the age at menopause and subsequent cardiovascular mortality, we studied a cohort of postmenopausal women aged 50-65 years at enrolment in an experimental breast cancer screening project in 1974-77; the women were followed up for a median of 16 years (range 1-20 years).

Patients and Methods

Patients

Between December, 1974, and September, 1977, 14,697 (72%) of the 20,555 women born between 1911 and 1925, living in the city of Utrecht, Netherlands, were enrolled in the DOM Project.[12] The breast cancer screening was repeated several times (maximum four; women dropped out between rounds). 2203 of the women were within a year of their last menstrual period and were deemed premenopausal. The remaining 12,494 reported that menses had ceased at least 12 months previously, and they were classified as postmenopausal. We excluded data for 1,004 of the 2,203 premenopausal women for whom the age at menopause could not be calculated from follow-up data, because they did not attend further screening sessions. Data for 1,199 women who became menopausal during follow-up were included in the analysis, starting from the year they became postmenopausal. Data for 1,578 women were excluded because of use of estrogen replacement therapy, and the self-reported age at menopause was probably not reliable. Thus, 12,115 women were included in the present analysis.

Municipal registries informed the Epidemiology Department each month about moves and deaths of cohort members. At the end of the follow-up period (Dec 31, 1994) 1,459 women (12% of the population) had moved outside the DOM area. The median follow-up for these women was 10 years, with a maximum of 20 years (whole cohort median 16, maximum 20 years). Cause of death was ascertained from the women's general practitioners. During the 20 years of follow-up, 2,022 women died, 824 of cardiovascular diseases, 726 of cancer, 94 from injury or external causes, including accidents and suicides, and 378 from other causes.

Questionnaires on menopausal status, age at menopause, medication use, cardiovascular risk factors, and indicators of ovarian function were completed at each screening visit.

Menopause was defined as cessation of menstrual bleeding for at least 12 months. Hypertension was defined as systolic blood pressure of 160 mmHg or more, diastolic blood pressure of 90 mmHg or more, use of antihypertensive medication, or a combination of these features. Women were classified as diabetic if they reported use of oral hypoglycaemic drugs or insulin or were on a diabetes diet. In the original questionnaire, previous or present cardiovascular disease was recorded as ischaemic cerebral attacks or myocardial infarction up to 5 years before the second screening visit or use of medication for cardiovascular diseases.

This medication consisted of aminoglycosides, antiarrhythmic drugs, nitrates, other antianginal drugs, or anticoagulants. Oral contraceptive use was coded as never use or ever use in statistical analyses, since the number of the women taking oral contraceptives was too small for detailed analysis. Parity and age at first delivery were classified in three categories—no children, children before or at age

24, and children after age 24. Height, weight, and subscapular and triceps skinfold thicknesses were measured at the first screening visit. Body-mass index was calculated and dichotomised at 30 kg/mm or more. Skinfold thicknesses were measured with callipers that could not measure skinfolds thicker than 40 mm, so such skinfolds were coded as 40 mm on the original registration forms. The study population was divided into subgroups by quintiles of subscapular as well as triceps skinfolds, resulting in subgroups of women with equally distributed fat, peripheral obesity, and upper-body obesity, respectively.[13]

Total cholesterol was measured in a sample of the population (2,179). Blood pressure measurements started only after the first 961 women had been screened, and are thus missing for those women. This subgroup was large enough for these data to be included as a separate category of the hypertension variable in statistical analyses. Data on smoking and previous cardiovascular diseases were collected at the second screening visit, 15 years after the first visit, and are therefore not known for women who did not attend the second screening (2,458). These data are also considered as separate categories in the statistical analysis.

The endpoint of the analysis was total cardiovascular mortality, codes 390-459 of the International Classification of Diseases, Ninth Revision (ICD-9). Death from other causes, loss to follow-up due to moving outside the DOM area, and withdrawal from the study were censoring events.

The association of age at menopause and cardiovascular mortality was first assessed by annual hazard estimates for biological ages between 50 and 80.[14] Biological age was a continuous variable, and age at menopause was classified in five categories (<40, 40-44, 45-49, 50-54, >54). Annual hazards were smoothed with a bandwidth of 5 years, and 95% CI were calculated.

Cox regression analysis was used to quantify further the effect of age at menopause on cardiovascular mortality. Since biological age is a major risk factor for cardiovascular mortality, all analyses were adjusted for age. This adjustment was done with biological age as the time axis. Since age at entry varied between 50 and 65, we had to account for left truncation of the data caused by the staggered entry. Age at menopause was analyzed as a continuous variable, with the assumption of a linear relation between age at menopause and cardiovascular mortality.

This approach implies that a menopause delay of 1 year has identical effects over the entire range of menopause ages. We used a restricted cubic spline function of age at menopause with three knots to test the linearity assumption. The use of such a function has been proposed as a statistically efficient procedure to detect non-linearity.[15] The Cox model further assumes that the hazards are proportional over time.

Proportionality of the effect of age at menopause was examined graphically in a plot of the logarithm of the annual hazards and was statistically tested by the addition to the Cox model of the interaction term of age at menopause and biological age. Because age at entry varied between 50 and 65, a cohort effect may have confounded the association at issue. This was approximated by year of birth. To study whether year of birth or other known cardiovascular risk factors caused confounding, we entered them first individually and then simultaneously into the Cox model with age at menopause to see whether the crude hazard ratio of age at menopause changed substantially. The effects of age at menopause were investigated in predetermined subgroups: women with different types of menopause (natural, hysterectomy, oophorectomy, radiation/surgery type unknown), and smokers and non-smokers. To test the significance of the subgroup effects, interaction terms of age at menopause with type of menopause and smoking were added to the Cox model, respectively.

Results

Baseline characteristics were distributed similarly among the strata of age at menopause. Oral contraceptive use was rare among these women, who were aged 37-52 when oral contraceptives were introduced in the Netherlands.

The risk of cardiovascular mortality was higher at all three biological ages analyzed for women who had early menopause. Each year that the menopause is delayed decreases the annual hazard of cardiovascular death by 2%. For example, a woman with menopause at age 45 has a risk of cardiovascular death 0.98 times that of a woman who has her menopause at age 44.

The effect of age at menopause on cardiovascular mortality was reasonably linear. This finding means that the difference in effect of age at menopause on cardiovascular mortality between each pair of two consecutive menopausal years is equal—i.e., a menopause delay of 1 year at age 40 has the same effect as a 1-year delay at age 50.

The extra risk of cardiovascular mortality due to early menopause seemed to decrease with increasing biological age, although the difference had borderline significance. The cardiovascular mortality risks clearly differed among the age at menopause subgroups at biological age 60, but they were more similar at age 80. The estimated effect of each year of delay in menopause is a reduction in annual hazard of 3% for a woman of biological age 65, 2% for a 70-year-old, 1% for a 75-year-old, and no reduction for an 80-year-old.

Individually, none of the baseline variables influenced the estimation of the average hazard ratio. For women who had undergone hysterectomy, age at menopause was not associated with cardiovascular mortality. By contrast, for those who had had oophorectomy the effect might be stronger, although the differences in these hazard ratios were not significant. The hazard ratio for age at menopause was 1.007 in smokers and 0.976 in non-smokers, although again this difference was not significant.

Discussion

Our results clearly show an increased risk of cardiovascular mortality for women who have early menopause. Biases may have led to incorrect effect estimates. Selection bias could have led to an underestimation. Women had to survive until at least age 50 to be invited for screening. Furthermore, they had to be healthy enough to attend screening. Women who later died of cardiovascular disease were more likely to withdraw between screening rounds. Thus, women attending the first screening were probably at lower cardiovascular risk. Reanalysis of the data including only women who attended at least the second screening round, however, gave similar results. Underestimation of the effect of early menopause due to selection bias will therefore be slight.

Although the study design was prospective, 85% of the women were already postmenopausal at enrollment, which could lead to misclassification bias. Age at menopause as reported at the first screening round was compared with that reported in the fifth round, 7.5 years later, in a sample of 4,892 women. For 80% of the sample the two reports differed by at most 1 year; thus, misclassification was limited. The findings are similar to those of the Nurses' Health Study.[16]

Biased reporting and measurement of risk factors by women with an early menopause is an unlikely explanation for our results. Associations of type of menopause, parity and age at first delivery, oral contraceptive use, smoking behavior, and body-mass index with age at menopause have been reported previously.[17-20] Hypertension, total cholesterol, body-fat distribution, presence of diabetes, and previous cardiovascular events are known risk factors for cardiovascular mortality. Adjustment for potential confounders was achieved by adding these factors individually or simultaneously into the Cox model. For parity we also checked whether the number of children was a potential confounder, and found that it was not. Information on lipoprotein fractions and subfractions was not available. However, since lipid concentrations are probably involved in the biological mechanism of the effect of estrogens on cardiovascular diseases, it would be inappropriate to adjust for lipid concentrations. Reanalysis of the data for women with complete data only gave similar results for the estimated hazard ratios. The possibility of ineffective adjustment caused by inclusion of missing data as separate categories of variables can therefore be excluded.

The effect of age at menopause on cardiovascular mortality was absent for women who had undergone hysterectomy and stronger for those who had had oophorectomy. This difference, although not statistically significant, is consistent with the postulated biological mechanism that hysterectomy does not lead to immediate cessation of estrogen production, whereas oophorectomy does.

Smoking advances the age of natural menopause by about 1.5 years.[21] The effect of age at menopause may be expected to differ between smokers and non-smokers, because smokers become menopausal even earlier. Although the effect of age at menopause in the various smoking subgroups did not differ significantly, the hazard ratio of age at menopause was almost unity for smoking women. The effect of smoking on cardiovascular mortality seems to be so strong as to over-ride the effect of an early menopause.

The evidence that reduced exposure to endogenous estrogens leads to increased cardiovascular morbidity has mainly come from studies of postmenopausal exogenous estrogen replacement,[6] for which a relative risk of 0.56 (95% CI 0.50-0.61) has been estimated.[22]

Morbidity and mortality statistics suggest that the decrease in the gap between cardiovascular morbidity and mortality in men and women cannot be attributed to the menopause.[9,23-25] Studies on the effect of endogenous estrogens on the occurrence of cardiovascular disease have been inconclusive.[2,5,26,27] The only prospective studies reported inconsistent results.[2,3] The Framingham Heart Study reported higher risk of cardiovascular disease in postmenopausal women that was even more pronounced in women aged 40-44 years,[2] whereas the Nurses' Health Study found no significant association with time since natural menopause.[3] In both cohorts, the women were young for cardiovascular disease to occur, less than 55 and 61 years old, respectively, and the time from menopause to cardiovascular disease may have been too short to allow convincing results to be shown. By contrast, in our study the oldest women were 85 years old and the postmenopausal follow-up extended to a maximum of 20 years.

The only investigation in which plasma concentrations of estrogens were measured did not show any association with cardiovascular mortality.[27] However, plasma concentrations were measured in post-menopausal women, and such measurements do not necessarily reflect premenopausal hormone concentrations.

In conclusion, our study provides evidence that early menopause is an independent risk factor for cardiovascular mortality and supports the hypothesis that reduced endogenous estrogen exposure increases cardiovascular mortality risk. The effect of an early menopause may be more important at younger biological ages.

The study was supported by grant 92.361 from the Netherlands Heart Foundation.

—by Yvonne T. van der Schouw, Yolanda van der Graaf,
Ewout W. Steyerberg, Marinus J.C. Eijkemans,
and Jan Dirk Banga.

References

1. Kannel WB, Hjortland MC, McNamara PM, Gordon T, Menopause and the risk of cardiovascular disease: the Framingham study. *Ann Intern Med* 1976; 85:447-52.

2. Gordon T, Kannel WB, Hjortland MC, McNamara PM, Menopause and coronary heart disease: the Framingham study. *Ann Intern Med* 1978; 89:151-61.

3. Colditz GA, Willett WC, Stampfer MJ, Rosner B, Speizer FE, Hennekens CH, Menopause and the risk of coronary heart disease in women. *N Engl J Med* 1987; 316:1105-10.

4. Parrish HM, Carr CA, Hall DG, King TM, Time interval from castration in premenopausal women to development of excessive coronary atherosclerisis. *Am J Obstet Gynecol* 1967; 99:155-62.

5. Robinson RW, Higano N, Cohen WD, Increased incidence of coronary heart disease in women castrated prior to the menopause. *Arch Intern Med* 1959; 104:908-13.

6. Barrett-Connor EL, Bush TL, Estrogen and coronary heart disease in women. *JAMA* 1991; 265:1861-67.

7. Wuest JH, Dry TJ, Edwards JE, The degree of coronary atherosclerosis in bilaterally oophorectomised women. *Circulation* 1953; 8:801-08.

8. Rivin AU, Dimitroff SP, The incidence and severity of cornary atherosclerosis in estrogen-treated males, and in females with a hypoestrogenic or a hyperestrogenic state. *Circulation* 1954; 9:533-39.

9. Winkelstein W, Stichever MA, Lilienfield AM, Occurrence of pregnancy, abortion and artificial menopause among women with coronary artery disease. *J Chron Dis* 1958; 7:273-86.

10. Bengtsson C, Rybo G, Westerberg H, Number of pregnancies, use of oral contraceptives and menopausal age in women with ischaemic heart disease, compared to a population sample of women. *Acta Med Scand* 1973; 89 (suppl):75-81.

11. Beard CM, Fuster V, Annegers JF, Reproductive history in women with coronary heart disease: a case control study. *Am J Epidemiol* 1984; 120:108-14.

12. Waard de F, Collette HJA, Rombach JJ, Baanders-van Halewijn EA, Honing C, The DOM project for early diagnosis of breast cancer. *J Chron Dis* 1984; 47:41-44.

13. Tonkelaar den I, Seidell JC, Collette HJA, Waard de F, A prospective study on obesity and subcutaneous fat patterning in relation to breast cancer in post-menopausal women participating in the DOM project. *Br J Cancer* 1994; 69:352-57.

14. Breslow NE, Day NE, Statistical methods in cancer research, volume II. The design and analysis of cohort studies. Oxford: *Oxford University Press*, 1987:195.

15. Harrell FE Jr, Lee KL, Pollock BG, Regression models in clinical studies: determining relationships between predictors and response. *J Natl Cancer Inst* 1985; 80:1198-202.

16. Colditz GA, Stampfer MJ, Willett WC, et al., Reproducibility and validity of self-reported menopausal status in a prospective cohort study. *Am J Epidemiol* 1987; 126:319-25.

17. Stanford JL, Hartge P, Brinton LA, Hoover RN, Brookmeyer R, Factors influencing the age at natural menopause. *J Chron Dis* 1987; 40:995-1002.

18. Midgette AS, Baron JA, Cigarette smoking and the risk of natural menopause. *Epidemiology* 1990; 1:474-80.

19. Luoto R, Kaprio J, Uutela A, Age at natural menopause and sociodemographic status in Finland. *Am J Epidemiol* 1994; 139:64-76.

20. Stampfer MJ, Colditz GA, Willett WC, Menopause and heart disease: a review. *Ann NY Acad Sci* 1990; 592:193-203.

21. Brambilla DJ, McKinlay SM, A prospective study of factors affecting age at menopause. *J Clin Epidemiol* 1989; 42:1031-39.

22. Stampfer MJ, Colditz GA, Estrogen replacement therapy and coronary heart disease: a quantitative assessment of the epidemiologic evidence. *Prev Med* 1991; 20:47-63.

23. Corrao JM, Becker RC, Ockene IS, Hamilton GA, Coronary heart disease risk factors in women. *Cardiology* 1990; 77 (suppl):8-24.

24. Tracey RE, Sex differences in coronary artery disease: two opposing views. *J Chron Dis* 1966; 19:1245-51.

25. Heller RF, Jacobs HS, Coronary heart disease in relation to age, sex, and the menopause. *BMJ* 1978; i:472-74.

26. Rosenberg L, Hennekens CH, Rosner B, Belanger C, Rothman KJ, Speizer FE, Early menopause and the risk of myocardial infarction. *Am J Obstet Gynecol* 1981; 139:47-51.

27. Barrett-Connor EL, Goodman-Gruen D, Prospective study of endogenous sex hormones and fatal cardiovascular disease in postmenopausal women. *BMJ* 1995; 311:1193-96.

Chapter 9

Depression Can Break Your Heart

Research over the past two decades has shown that depression and heart disease are common companions and what is worse, each can lead to the other. It appears now that depression is an important risk factor for heart disease along with high blood cholesterol and high blood pressure. In a study conducted in Baltimore, it was found that of 1,551 people who were free of heart disease those who were depressed were four times more likely to have a heart attack in the next 14 years than those who were not. Researchers in Montreal found that heart patients who were depressed were four times as likely to die in the next six months as those who were not depressed.

Depression may make it harder to take the medications needed and to carry out the treatment for heart disease. Depression may also result in chronically elevated levels of stress hormones, such as cortisol and adrenaline, and the activation of the sympathetic nervous system (part of the "fight or flight" response) which can have deleterious effects on the heart.

The first studies of heart disease and depression showed that people with heart disease were more depressed than healthy people. While about one in six people have an episode of major depression, the number goes to one in two for people with heart disease. Furthermore, other researchers have found that most heart patients are not

National Heart, Lung, and Blood Institute (NHLBI), NIH Publication No. 99-4592, revised June 1999; and "Depression: What Every Woman Should Know," an undated fact sheet produced by the National Institute of Mental Health (NIMH).

treated for depression. Doctors tend to miss the diagnosis of depression and even when they treat it they often treat it with sedatives which may make the depression worse.

The public health impact of depression and heart disease, both separately and together, is enormous. Depression is the estimated leading cause of disability worldwide, and heart disease is by far the leading cause of death in the United States. Approximately one in three of Americans will die of some form of heart disease.

Studies indicate that depression can appear after heart disease and/or heart disease surgery. In one investigation, nearly half of the patients studied one week after cardiopulmonary bypass surgery experienced serious cognitive problems, which may contribute to clinical depression in some patients.

There are also multiple studies indicating that heart disease can follow depression. Psychological distress may cause rapid heartbeat, high blood pressure, and faster blood clotting. It can also lead to elevated insulin and cholesterol levels. These risk factors, with obesity, form a constellation of symptoms and often serve as a predictor of and a response to heart disease. Depressed individuals may feel slowed down and still have high levels of stress hormones. This can increase the work of the heart. When patients are caught in a fight or flight reaction, the body's metabolism is diverted away from the type of tissue repair needed in heart disease.

Regardless of cause, the combination of depression and heart disease is associated with increased sickness and death making effective treatment of depression imperative. Pharmacological and cognitive-behavioral therapy treatments for depression are relatively well developed and play an important role in reducing the adverse impact of depression. With the advent of the selective serotonin reuptake inhibitors to treat depression, more medically ill patients can be treated without the complicating cardiovascular side effects of the previous drugs available. Ongoing research is investigating whether these treatments also reduce the associated risk of a second heart attack. Furthermore, preventive interventions based on cognitive-behavior theories of depression also merit attention as approaches for avoiding adverse outcomes associated with both disorders. These interventions may help promote adherence and behavior change that may increase the impact of available pharmacological and behavioral approaches to both diseases.

Exercise is another potential pathway to reducing both depression and heart disease. Exercise is related to fewer depressive symptoms in observational studies and appears to be as efficacious as psychotherapy in patients with mild depression. Exercise, of course, is a major protective factor against heart disease as well.

The NIMH and the National Heart, Lung and Blood Institute are invested in uncovering the complicated relationship between depression and heart disease. They support research on the basic mechanisms and processes linking co-morbid mental and medical disorders to identify potent, modifiable risk factors and protective processes amenable to medical and behavioral interventions that will reduce the adverse outcomes associated with both types of disorders.

Understanding Special Issues in Depression: A Woman's Guide to Its Diagnosis and Treatment

Life is full of emotional ups and downs. But when the "down" times are long lasting or interfere with an individual's ability to function, that person may be suffering from a common, serious illness—depression.

Clinical depression affects mood, mind, body, and behavior. Research has shown that in the United States more than 19 million people—almost one in ten adults—will experience depression this year, yet nearly two thirds will not get the help they need. Treatment can alleviate the symptoms in over 80 percent of the cases. Yet, because it often goes unrecognized, depression continues to cause unnecessary suffering.

Women are disproportionately affected by depression, experiencing it at roughly twice the rate of men. Research continues to explore how the illness affects women. At the same time, it is important to increase women's awareness of what is already known about depression, so that they seek early and appropriate treatment.

To grasp the specifics of depression in women, it is essential to have a broad understanding of the illness itself. To this end, this chapter presents an overview of depression as a pervasive and impairing illness that affects women and men in similar fashion. It then focuses on special issues—biological, life cycle, and psychosocial—that are unique to women and may be associated with depression.

What Is "Depression"?

There are three types of depression:

1. Major depression, also known as unipolar or clinical depression, people have some or all of the symptoms (listed in the

following section) for at least 2 weeks or as long as several months or even longer. Episodes of the illness can occur once, twice, or several times in a lifetime.

2. In dysthymia, the same symptoms are present though milder, but lasting at least two years. People with dysthymia also can experience major depressive episodes, which is sometimes called a "double depression."

3. Manic-depression, or bipolar illness, which is not nearly as common as other forms of depressive illness each year, and involves disruptive cycles of depressive symptoms that alternate with euphoria, irritable excitement or mania.

The Symptoms of Depression and Mania

A thorough diagnostic evaluation is needed if five or more of the following symptoms persist for more than two weeks, or if they interfere with work or family life. An evaluation involves a complete physical checkup and information-gathering on family health history.

Not everyone with depression experiences each of these symptoms. The severity of the symptoms also varies from person to person.

Depression

- Persistent sad, anxious, or "empty" mood
- Loss of interest or pleasure in activities, including sex
- Restlessness, irritability, or excessive crying
- Feelings of guilt, worthlessness, helplessness, hopelessness, pessimism
- Sleeping too much or too little, early-morning awakening
- Appetite and/or weight loss or overeating and weight gain
- Decreased energy, fatigue, feeling "slowed down"
- Thoughts of death or suicide, or suicide attempts
- Difficulty concentrating, remembering, or making decisions
- Persistent physical symptoms that do not respond to treatment, such as headaches, digestive disorders, and chronic pain

Mania

- Abnormally elevated mood

- Irritability
- Severe insomnia
- Grandiose notions
- Increased talking
- Racing thoughts
- Increased activity, including sexual activity
- Markedly increased energy
- Poor judgement that leads to risk-taking behavior
- Inappropriate social behavior

Some people mistakenly try to "reduce their" depressive symptoms through alcohol or other mood-altering drugs, while such drugs may provide temporary relief, they will eventually complicate the depressive disorder and its treatment, and can lead to dependence and the life problems that come with it.

Women Are at Greater Risk for Depression Than Men

Major depression and dysthymia affect twice as many women as men. This two-to-one ratio exists regardless of racial and ethnic background or economic status. The same ratio has been reported in eleven other countries all over the world. Men and women have about the same rate of bipolar disorder (manic depression), though its course in women typically has more depressive and fewer manic episodes. Also, a greater number of women have the rapid cycling form of bipolar disorder, which may be more resistant to standard treatments.

A variety of factors unique to women's lives are suspected to play a role in developing depression. Research is focused on understanding these, including: reproductive, hormonal, genetic or other biological factors; abuse and oppression; interpersonal factors; and certain psychological and personality characteristics. And yet, the specific causes of depression in women remain unclear; many women exposed to these factors do not develop depression. What is clear is that regardless of the contributing factors, depression is a highly treatable illness and that the types of treatment discussed later in this chapter are effective for a majority of women.

The Many Dimensions of Depression in Women

Investigators are focusing on the following areas in their study of depression in women:

77

The Issues of Adolescence

Studies show that the higher incidence of depression in females begins in adolescence, when roles and expectations change dramatically. The stresses of adolescence include forming an identity, confronting sexuality, separating from parents, and making decisions for the first time, along with other physical, intellectual, and hormonal changes. These stresses are generally different for boys and girls, and may be associated more often with depression in females.

Adulthood: Relationships and Work Roles

It is known that stress in general can contribute to depression in persons biologically vulnerable to the illness. Some have theorized that higher incidence of depression in women is not due to greater vulnerability, but to the particular stresses that many women face. These stresses include major responsibilities at home and work, single parenthood, and caring for children and aging parents, and are areas currently under study. How these factors may uniquely effect women is not yet fully understood.

Reproductive Events

Women's reproductive events include the menstrual cycle, pregnancy, the postpregnancy period, infertility, menopause, and sometimes, the decision not to have children. These events bring fluctuations in mood that for some women include depression. Researchers have confirmed that hormones have an effect on the brain chemistry that controls emotions and mood; a specific biological mechanism explaining hormonal involvement is not known, however.

Many women experience certain behavioral and physical changes associated with phases of their menstrual cycles. In some women, these changes are severe, occur regularly, and include depressed feelings, irritability, and other emotional and physical changes. Called premenstrual syndrome, its relation to depressive disorders is not yet understood. Some have questioned whether it is, in fact, a disorder. Further research will no doubt add to our understanding of this long-ignored condition.

Postpartum depressions can range from transient "blues" following childbirth to severe, incapacitating, psychotic depressions. Studies suggest that women who experience depression after childbirth very often have had prior depressive episodes. However, for most women, postpartum depressions are transient, with no adverse consequences.

Pregnancy (if it is desired) seldom contributes to depression, and having an abortion does not appear to lead to a higher incidence of depression. Women with infertility problems may be subject to extreme anxiety or sadness, though it is unclear if this contributes to a higher rate of depressive illness. In addition, young motherhood may be a time of heightened risk for depression, due to the stress and demands it imposes.

Personality and Psychology

Studies indicate that individuals with certain characteristics—pessimistic thinking, low self-esteem, a sense of having little control over life events, and proneness to excessive worrying—are more likely to develop depression. These attributes may heighten the effect of stressful events or interfere with taking action to cope with them. Some experts have suggested that the traditional upbringing of girls might foster these traits and that may be a factor in the higher rate of depression.

Others have suggested that women are not more vulnerable to depression than men, but simply express or label their symptoms differently. Women may be more likely to admit feelings of depression, brood about their feelings, or seek professional assistance. Men, on the other hand, may be socially conditioned to deny such feelings or to bury them in alcohol, as reflected in the higher rates of alcoholism in men. Current research may provide some answers about which of these theories is correct.

Victimization

Studies show that women molested as children are more likely to have clinical depression at some time in their lives than those with no such history. In addition, several studies show a higher incidence of depression among women who were raped as adults. Since far more women than men were sexually abused as children, these findings are relevant. Women who experience other commonly occurring forms of abuse, such as physical abuse and sexual harassment on the job, also may experience higher rates of depression. Abuse may lead to depression by fostering low self-esteem, a sense of helplessness, self-blame, and social isolation. At present, more research is needed to understand whether victimization is connected specifically to depression.

Poverty

Women and children represent seventy-five percent of the U.S. population considered poor. Some researchers are therefore exploring the possibility that poverty is one of the "pathways to depression." Low economic status brings with it many stresses, including isolation, uncertainty, frequent negative events, and poor access to helpful resources. Sadness and low morale are more common among persons with low incomes and those lacking social supports. But research has not yet established whether depressive illnesses are more prevalent among those facing environmental stressors such as these. One very large study has shown that these illnesses tend to equally effect the poor and the rich.

Depression in Later Adulthood

Once, depression at menopause was considered a unique illness known as "involutional melancholia." Research has shown, however, that depressive illnesses are no different, and no more likely to occur, at menopause than at other ages. In fact, the women most vulnerable to change-of-life depression are those with a history of past depressive episodes. An old theory, the "empty nest syndrome", stated that when children leave home, women may experience a profound loss of purpose and identity that leads to depression. However, studies show no increase in depressive illness among women at this stage of life.

As with younger age groups, more elderly women than men suffer from depressive illness. Similarly, for all age groups, being unmarried (which includes widowhood) is also a risk factor for depression. Despite this, depression should not be dismissed as a normal consequence of the physical, social and economic problems of later life. In fact, studies show that most older people feel satisfied with their lives.

About 800,000 persons are widowed each year, most of them are older, female, and experience varying degrees of depressive symptomatology. Most do not need formal treatment, but those who are moderately or severely sad appear to benefit from self-help groups or various psychosocial treatments. Remarkably, a third of widows/widowers meet criteria for major depressive episode in the first month after the death, and half of these remain clinically depressed 1 year later. These depressions respond to standard antidepressant medications, although there is relatively little research on when

80

to start medications or how medications should be combined with psychosocial treatments.

Depression Is a Treatable Illness

Even severe depression can be highly responsive to treatment. Indeed, believing one's condition is "incurable" is often part of the hopelessness that accompanies serious depression. Such patients should be provided with the information about the effectiveness of modern treatments for depression. As with many illnesses, the earlier treatment begins, the more effective and the greater the likelihood of preventing serious recurrences. Of course, treatment will not eliminate life's inevitable stresses and ups and downs. But it can greatly enhance the ability to manage such challenges and lead to greater enjoyment of life.

As a first step, a thorough physical examination may be recommended to rule out any physical illnesses that may cause depressive symptoms.

Types of Treatment for Depression

The most commonly used treatments for depression are antidepressant medication, psychotherapy, or a combination of the two. Which of these is the right treatment for an individual case and depends on the nature and severity of the depression and, to some extent, on individual preference. In mild or moderate depression, one or both of these treatments may be useful, while in severe or incapacitating depression, medication is generally recommended as a first step in the treatment. In combined treatment, medication can relieve physical symptoms quickly, while psychotherapy allows the opportunity to learn more effective ways of handling problems.

Medications

The medications used to treat depression include tricyclic antidepressants, monoamine oxidase inhibitors (MAOIs), serotonin reuptake inhibitors (SRIs), and bupropion. Each acts on different chemical pathways of the human brain related to moods. Antidepressant medications are not habit-forming. To be effective, medications must be taken for about 4-6 months (in a first episode), carefully following the doctor's instructions. Medications must be monitored to ensure the most effective dosage and to minimize side effects.

The prescribing doctor will provide information about possible side-effects and dietary restrictions. In addition, other medically prescribed medications being used should be reviewed because some can interact negatively with antidepressant medication. There may be restrictions during pregnancy.

Psychotherapy

In mild to moderate cases, psychotherapy is also a treatment option. Some short-term (10-20 week) therapies have been very effective in several types of depression. "Talking" therapies help patients gain insight into and resolve their problems through verbal give-and-take with the therapist. "Behavioral" therapies help patients learn new behaviors that lead to more satisfaction in life, and "unlearn" counter-productive behaviors.

Research has shown that two short-term psychotherapies, Interpersonal and Cognitive/Behavioral, are helpful for some forms of depression. Interpersonal therapy works to change interpersonal relationships that cause or exacerbate depression. Cognitive/Behavioral therapy helps change negative styles of thinking and behaving that may contribute to the depression.

Other Treatments

Despite the unfavorable publicity electroconvulsive therapy (ECT) has received, research has shown that there are circumstances in which its use is medically justified and can even save lives. This is particularly true for those with extreme suicide risk, psychotic agitation, severe weight loss or physical debilitation due to other physical illness. ECT may also be recommended for persons who cannot take or do not respond to medication.

Some people experience depressive illness during the winter (seasonal depression), and are helped by a new form of therapy using lights, called phototherapy.

Treating Recurrent Depression

Even when treatment is successful, depression may recur. Studies indicate that certain treatment strategies are very useful in this instance. Continuation of antidepressant medication at the same dose that successfully treated the acute episode can often prevent recurrence. Monthly interpersonal psychotherapy can lengthen the time between episodes in patients not taking medication.

The Path to Healing

Reaping the benefits of treatment begins by recognizing the signs of depression. The next step is to be evaluated by a qualified professional. Depression can be diagnosed and treated by primary care physicians as well as psychiatrists, psychologists, clinical social workers, and other mental health professionals.

Treatment is a partnership between the patient and the health care provider. An informed consumer knows her treatment options, and discusses concerns with her provider as they arise. If there are no positive results after 2-3 months of treatment, or if symptoms worsen, discuss another treatment approach with the provider. Getting a second opinion from another health or mental health professional may also be in order.

Here, again, are the steps to healing:

- Check your symptoms against the list.

- Talk to a health or mental health professional.

- Choose a treatment professional and a treatment approach.

- Consider yourself a partner in treatment, and be an informed consumer.

- If you are not comfortable or satisfied after about 2-3 months, discuss this with your provider. Different or additional treatment may be recommended.

- If you experience a recurrence, remember what you know about coping with depression, and don't shy away from seeking help again.

For Additional Information about Depression Write To:

Depression
6001 Executive Boulevard
Room 8184, MSC 9663
Bethesda, MD 20892-9663
For free brochures on depression and its treatment, call: 1-800-421-4211

For More Information About National Institute of Mental Health (NIMH)

The Office of Communications and Public Liaison carries out educational activities and publishes and distributes research reports, press releases, fact sheets, and publications intended for researchers, health care providers, and the general public. A publications list may be obtained on the web at http://www.nimh.nih.gov/publist/puborder.cfm or by contacting:

Office of Communications and Public Liaison, NIMH
Information Resources and Inquiries Branch
6001 Executive Blvd
Room 8184, MSC 9663
Bethesda, MD 20892-9663
Phone: 301-443-4513
Fax: 301-443-4279
Mental Health FAX4U: 301-443-5158
E-mail: nimhinfo@nih.gov
NIMH home page address: http://www.nimh.nih.gov

For information about NIMH and its programs, please email, write or phone us.

NIMH Public Inquiries
6001 Executive Boulevard, Rm. 8184, MSC 9663
Bethesda, MD 20892-9663 U.S.A.
Voice (301) 443-4513
Fax (301) 443-4279

Chapter 10

The Female Heart Patient and High LDL Cholesterol

A majority of women with coronary heart disease may have high levels of "bad cholesterol," even if they're taking lipid-lowering drugs, according to the April 23/30 *JAMA*. Helmut G. Schrott, MD, of the University of Iowa, Iowa City, and colleagues looked at 2,743 postmenopausal women with CHD who took part in the Heart and Estrogen/Progestin Replacement Study.

The researchers wanted to know how many of the volunteers met the guidelines recommended by the National Cholesterol Education Program's Adult Treatment Panel for low-density lipoprotein cholesterol.

They found: "Although 47% of participants were taking a lipid-lowering medication, 63% did not meet the 1988 treatment goal ... and 91% did not meet the 1993 goal." The researchers also found that higher LDL-C levels seemed to be associated with a higher body mass index, and with a diagnosis of CHD made before 1990. Lower LDL-C levels were associated with lipid-lowering treatment, never having been married, postgraduate education, and participation in both a regular exercise program and regular walking. Interestingly, hypertension, insulin-requiring diabetes and a history of gall bladder disease also were associated with having LDL cholesterol levels at or lower than the recommendation.

The women in the study ranged in age from 44 to 79; 88.7% were white; 7.9% were African-American; 2.0% were Hispanic; and the rest

American Medical News, May 5, 1997, Vol. 40, No. 17, Pg. 17(1), © 1997 American Medical Association; reprinted with permission.

belonged to other ethnic and racial groups. They were recruited at 18 centers across the United States from February 1993 to September 1994. The women were generally sedentary and overweight; 13.1% were current smokers; 49% were former smokers; 59.5% reported hypertension; and 23% had diabetes.

A total of 1,733 of the women in the study were either taking lipid-lowering therapy or met guidelines to receive drug therapy. The researchers found: "Nonuse of drug therapy was positively associated with African-American race/ethnicity, higher BMI, amount of alcohol consumption, current smoking, and CHD before 1985." They point out that other factors may account for some of the associations they found: "For members of the African-American community, reduced access to medical care and the higher cost of lipid-lowering medication may pose a barrier."

The researchers cite information showing that CHD is the most frequent cause of death among women. The prognosis for women is equal to or worse than for men following heart attack, coronary artery bypass grafting or angioplasty. Contributing factors may include the more frequent occurrence of other known coronary risk factors such as hypertension, diabetes, abnormal lipid levels, and perhaps the low-estrogen postmenopausal state itself.

Treating Hypercholesterolemia

In an accompanying editorial, Thomas A. Pearson, MD, PhD, formerly of the Mary Imogene Bassett Research Institute of Cooperstown, N.Y., currently with the University of Rochester School of Medicine, and Merle Myerson, MD, EdD, of the Mary Imogene Bassett Research Institute applaud Dr. Schrott and his colleagues for pointing out the underutilization of lipid-lowering drugs to reduce recurrence, disability and death in women with CHD. They also cite two additional studies, both suggesting that women may benefit more than men from lipid-lowering therapy. They write: "While not proving better efficacy of cholesterol-lowering treatment in women vs. men, these data certainly suggest that women with CHD should be treated as aggressively as men for elevated LDL cholesterol levels."

Chapter 11

Are Cholesterol Lowering Drugs Right for Women?

The first commercial ran on television just after Labor Day and was as direct as it was mysterious. Heart disease has killed more Americans than all of our wars combined, it said. It's time to fight back.

The spot directed viewers to look to their Sunday newspapers. There, full-page advertisements announced that a prescription drug called Pravachol was "the first and only cholesterol-lowering drug of its kind proven to help prevent first heart attacks."

The ad campaign, mounted by Bristol-Myers Squibb, was note-worthy for a number of reasons. It marked the first time that cholesterol-lowering drugs were advertised directly to consumers as preventive medicine. The marketing effort came just months after the Food and Drug Administration approved Pravachol for that use, spurred by a project known as the West of Scotland (or WestScot) study. Its results showed that the drug lowered the risk of death—even in men who had never been diagnosed with heart disease. Following nearly 6,600 Scottish men with moderately high cholesterol for five years, researchers found that the drug cut both cholesterol levels and overall mortality by about 20 percent. Reviewers at the FDA were not alone in finding the results persuasive; heart researchers also have been impressed.

Perhaps just as significantly, the advertisements left the impression that anyone with high cholesterol, women as well as men, might benefit from such drugs. But the WestScot study is most compelling for what it says about men, particularly men at very high risk for heart disease. "Clearly the trial had nothing to do with women," says David Atkins, a science adviser to the U.S. Preventive Services Task Force. "It was on Scottish men who were well into middle age. Many of them smoked, and anyone who's ever been to Scotland knows that the diet is pretty horrendous. There is a danger in saying that an average American man whose cholesterol is elevated has anything near the risk of the men in this study. And when it comes to the average woman, we're really in the dark."

"The good news is that these drugs are very effective. The question is, When is your risk of heart disease high enough to justify taking them?"

For women, the answer is very different than for men. After decades during which doctors and public health officials largely ignored the female heart, they have finally begun to pay attention. But that heightened awareness may have a downside. Women may be worrying more than they need to, especially when it comes to the danger posed by cholesterol.

Relatively little research exists on the subject of women and cholesterol. In a sense, women have been shortchanged by their good fortune. While heart disease is their number one killer—a fact that has received much play in the press lately—women tend to develop heart disease considerably later than men do. Men are hit hardest in their fifties and sixties, according to Harvard University epidemiologist JoAnn Manson, while women who succumb are usually at least in their seventies. The average woman of 45 or 50 has an extremely low risk of dying of heart disease during her next 20 years, says Manson, even if she has abnormally high cholesterol levels.

This difference means it is a good deal harder to gauge whether women might benefit from drugs that lower cholesterol. The WestScot scientists purposely chose men at high risk so that a relatively large number of heart attacks would be likely over the five years of the study, says researcher Judith Walsh of the University of California at San Francisco, who has studied women and cholesterol. That way, if Pravachol cut that number significantly, the improvement would be both noticeable and scientifically meaningful. But with women, the researchers would have had to study tens of thousands to get the same degree of certainty.

Why women are less prone to heart disease seems to have little to do with lifestyle and much to do with biology. Over the past few years researchers have pinpointed a number of ways in which estrogen benefits women's hearts and arteries. The hormone appears to lower levels of the blood proteins required for clotting, which sometimes clog up arteries as well. It also seems to relax arteries, allowing them to stretch to maintain blood flow if a partial blockage forms.

Perhaps most important, estrogen lowers levels of low-density lipoprotein, the type of cholesterol that can build up on artery walls to cause heart disease, and increases levels of high-density lipoprotein, which carts the bad stuff away from artery walls and back to the liver for disposal. Women have higher levels of HDL than men throughout life and lower levels of LDL until menopause.

Because of these advantages, total cholesterol is a less meaningful number for women than for men, say specialists on female heart disease. According to the National Cholesterol Education Program, a woman's cholesterol is high if it's over 240 milligrams per deciliter. But her risk of heart disease may nevertheless be low if much of that is HDL, says epidemiologist Walter Willett, codirector of the 20-year, 121,000-woman Nurses Health Study at Harvard. Cholesterol numbers needn't worry a woman unless her HDL is below 40 or her total cholesterol is more than five times her HDL—if, for instance, her total is 240 and her HDL is only 45.

Even then, a woman should heed the advice long given to men: Consider cholesterol drugs only after adding exercise to your daily routine and cutting back on meat, cheese, and other foods high in saturated fat. And keep those cholesterol numbers in perspective. Cholesterol is just one risk factor for heart disease, says Walsh, and for women, as for men, other factors weigh at least as heavily—a smoking habit, being sedentary or overweight, advancing age, illnesses such as diabetes, and a family history of heart disease.

Take a 45-year-old woman whose cholesterol is 260 but who has no other risk factors, says Walsh. She's not a good candidate for cholesterol-lowering drugs. After all, her chances of having a heart attack will remain very low for at least a couple of decades. These drugs are expensive and—like any medicine—carry risks, such as the small possibility of affecting liver function. Cholesterol-lowering medications of the sort used in WestScot, collectively known as statins, have proved extremely safe, but the studies have lasted only five to ten years.

"If you start a 45-year-old woman with high cholesterol on this drug to prevent her heart attack at 75," says Walsh, "what do we know about the risks of her taking this drug for 30 years? The answer is nothing."

Drug therapy clearly does make sense for women who already have heart disease; studies show that such women are helped as much by the drugs as men are. Because of the WestScot study, many researchers believe that some healthy women with high cholesterol may eventually prove to benefit from the drugs as well. But those women will probably be older and at higher risk than their male counterparts.

The point is to treat cholesterol with respect—and to treat cholesterol-lowering drugs the same way, says Atkins. "What I've seen is that women are sometimes treated with drugs when their risk really is not bad. My mother-in-law was told to change her diet because her total cholesterol reading was 260. Her levels of good cholesterol put her in the lowest possible risk category—she had nothing to gain from the changes she made. Another doctor could easily have put her on drugs if he wasn't paying attention."

—by Gary Taubes

Chapter 12

Reducing High Blood Cholesterol

High blood cholesterol is a condition that greatly increases your chances of developing coronary heart disease. That is because extra cholesterol in the blood settles on the inner walls of the arteries, narrowing them, allowing less blood to pass through them to the heart.

Today, about one-quarter of American women have blood cholesterol levels high enough to pose a serious risk for heart disease. Blood cholesterol among women tends to rise sharply beginning at about age 40 and continues to increase until about age 60.

Types of Cholesterol and Heart Disease Risk

The higher your total blood cholesterol level, the higher your heart disease risk. For all adults, a desirable total blood cholesterol level is less than 200 mg/dL. A level of 240 or above is considered high blood cholesterol. But even levels in the "borderline-high" category (200-239) boost the risk of heart disease.

Your level of high density lipoprotein, or HDL, also affects heart disease risk. If your HDL level is less than 35, your risk of heart disease goes up. Ask your health professional to check your total blood cholesterol and your HDL levels once every five years.

Your level of low density lipoprotein, or LDL, also affects risk. An LDL level below 130 is desirable, while levels of 130-159 are "borderline-high." LDL levels of 160 or above mean you have a high risk of

National Heart, Lung, and Blood Institute (NHLBI), NIH Publication No. 96-3658, reprinted September 1996.

developing coronary heart disease. While an LDL measurement is not necessary for your first cholesterol test, your doctor may recommend that you have your LDL levels checked after reviewing your initial test results and your medical history. Lowering LDL-cholesterol is the main goal of treatment.

Lowering Your Blood Cholesterol

Reducing your blood cholesterol level can greatly lessen the chances of developing coronary heart disease. Most people can lower their blood cholesterol by changing their diet, losing excess weight, and increasing physical activity.

Changing Your Eating Habits

To lower your blood cholesterol through diet, eat fewer foods high in saturated fat, total fat, and cholesterol. The total fat in your diet should average no more than 30 percent of your calories. Your "fat allowance" should be divided tip this way:

- Saturated fat should make up 8 to 10 percent of total calories.

- A Polyunsaturated fat should not be more than 10 percent of total calories.

- Monounsaturated fat should make up 10 to 15 percent of total calories.

In addition, you should eat less than 300 mg of cholesterol per day. If you follow these guidelines for about 6 months and your blood cholesterol does not drop to a goal level set for you by your doctor, you may need to cut back still more on saturated fat and cholesterol.

Fat Finding

Now, let's get practical. Which foods belong to which categories.

Saturated fat is found mainly in foods that come from animals. Whole milk dairy products such as butter, cheese, milk, and ice cream all contain high amounts of saturated fat. The fat in meat and poultry skin is also high in saturated fat. A few vegetable fats—coconut oil, cocoa butter, palm kernel oil, and palm oil—are also high in saturated fat.

Remember: Saturated fat boosts your blood cholesterol level more than anything else in your diet. Eating fewer foods high in saturated fat is the best way to lower your blood cholesterol level.

Unsaturated fat helps to lower cholesterol levels when you use it in place of saturated fat. One type is polyunsaturated fat, which is found in many cooking and salad oils, and in margarine, especially liquid and soft varieties. Another type is monounsaturated fat, which is found in olive and canola oils.

Cholesterol is found only in foods that come from animals. Egg yolks and organ meats (such as liver) are very high in cholesterol.

Now You're Cooking

Planning meals aimed at reducing blood cholesterol doesn't have to be complicated. Here are a few suggestions:

- Choose fish, poultry, and lean cuts of meat, and remove the fat and skin before eating. Eat no more than about 6 ounces per day.

- Broil, bake, roast, or poach foods rather than fry them.

- Cut down on high fat processed meats, including sausage, bacon, and such cold cuts as salami and bologna.

- Limit organ meats such as liver, kidney, or brains.

- Use skim or low fat milk and cheeses, and low or nonfat yogurt.

- Instead of butter, use liquid or soft margarine or vegetable oils high in unsaturated fats. Use all fats and oils sparingly.

- Eat egg yolks only in moderation. Egg whites contain no fat or cholesterol and can be eaten often.

- Eat plenty of fruits and vegetables, as well as cereals, breads, rice, and pasta made from enriched or whole grains (for example, rye bread or whole wheat spaghetti).

- Many packaged and processed foods are high in saturated fats. Get in the habit of reading food labels. Look for the "Nutrition Facts" on the label and choose products that are lowest in fat and saturated fat. Also read product labels for cholesterol content.

Losing Weight

If you are overweight, losing weight also can help to lower high blood cholesterol, especially LDL cholesterol, and also may help boost

HDL levels. Choose a wide variety of low-calorie, nutritious foods in moderate amounts. If you have a lot of weight to lose, ask your doctor or a nutritionist to help you develop a sensible, well-balanced plan for gradual weight loss. Avoid fad diets and diet pills, because many cause troublesome side effects and none of them works for long-term weight loss.

Getting Physical

Regular physical activity can also help you improve your cholesterol "profile." Even low- to moderate-intensity activity, if done daily, can provide benefits. Examples of such activity are pleasure walking, gardening, yard work, moderate-to-heavy housework, dancing, and home exercise.

More vigorous exercise can raise HDL-cholesterol levels and also will improve the overall fitness of your heart. This kind of activity is called "aerobic" and includes jogging, swimming, jumping rope, or brisk walking or bicycling.

Regardless of the type of choose, be sure to activity you build up your activity level gradually over a period of several weeks. Also, check with your doctor first if you have any health problems, or if you are over 50 and are not used to energetic activity and plan a fairly strenuous program.

Medication

If you make the changes in your diet and lifestyle described above and your LDL-cholesterol levels still remain quite high, your doctor may also suggest that you take cholesterol-lowering medications. This recommendation also will depend on whether you have any other risk factors for coronary heart disease.

If you have not yet gone through menopause, you should not be prescribed cholesterol-lowering drugs unless your cholesterol level is extremely high, you have heart disease or other risk factors for heart disease or you have a strong family history of early heart disease. If you have gone through menopause, your doctor may prescribe an estrogen medicine to help lower your cholesterol levels before recommending a cholesterol-lowering drug.

If your doctor does prescribe medicines, you must also continue your cholesterol lowering diet because the combination may allow you to take less medicine. Always try to lower your cholesterol levels with diet and other lifestyle changes before adding medication.

Table 12.1. Blood Cholesterol Levels

	Desirable	Borderline-High	High
Total Cholesterol	less than 200 mg/dL	200-239 mg/dL	240 mg/dL and above
LDL Cholesterol	less than 130 mg/dL	130-159 mg/dL	160 mg/dL and above
HDL Cholesterol	a low HDL cholesterol is less dm 35 mg/dL		

Table 12.2. Figuring Out Fat

Your personal "fat allowance" depends on how many calories you take in each day. Remember, the total fat in your diet should average no more than 30 percent of your calories, and saturated fat should be no more than 10 percent. Table 12.2 shows the upper limit on total fat and saturated fat grams you should eat, depending on how many calories you consume each day. Check food labels to find out the number of fat grams (total and saturated) in each serving.

Total Calories (per day)	Total Fat* (in grams)	Saturated Fat** (in grams)
1,500	50	15
1,800	60	18
2,000	65	20
2,500	80	25

*Amounts are equal to 30 percent of total calories (rounded down to the nearest 5); the recommendation is to eat this much or less.

**Amounts are equal to 9 percent of total calories; the recommendation is to eat less than 10 percent of total calories as saturated fat. Each gram of fat is equal to 9 calories.

Note: On average, women consume about 1,800 calories a day, and men consume about 2,500 calories a day.

Table 12.3. The Healthy Diet: Back to Basics

Food Group	Daily Servings	What Counts As A Serving
vegetables	3-5 servings	1 cup raw leafy greens 1/2 cup other vegetables
fruits	2-4 servings	1 medium apple, banana, orange 1/2 cup fruit—fresh, cooked, canned 3/4 cup juice
breads, cereals, rice, and pasta	6-11 servings	1 slice bread 1/2 bun or bagel 1 ounce dry cereal 1/2 cup cooked cereal, rice, pasta
milk, yogurt, and cheese	2-3 servings	1 cup milk (skim or low fat) 8 ounces low fat yogurt 1 1/2 ounces low fat natural cheese 2 ounces low fat processed cheese
meat, poultry, fish, and dry peas and beans, eggs, and nuts	2-3 servings	This totals 6 ounces of cooked lean meat, poultry without skin, or fish per day Count 1/2 cup cooked beans, 1 egg, or 2 Tbsp. peanut butter as 1 ounce meat (Limit the use of egg yolks and organ meats since they are high in cholesterol.)

Source: *Dietary Guidelines for Americans*, U.S. Department of Agriculture/ U.S. Department of Health and Human Services, 1990.

A Word about Margarine

You may have heard that margarine has a type of unsaturated fat called "trans" fat. "Trans" fats appear to raise blood cholesterol more than other unsaturated fats, but not as much as saturated fats. "Trans" fats are formed when vegetable oil is hardened to become margarine or shortening through a process called "hydrogenation." The harder the margarine or shortening, the more hydrogenated or saturated it is and the more "trans" fat it has. So buy soft or liquid margarine for spreading or cooking. Also, choose those containing liquid vegetable oil as the first ingredient.

Chapter 13

Preventing and Controlling High Blood Pressure

High blood pressure, or hypertension, greatly increases your chance of developing heart disease and is the most important risk factor for stroke. Even slightly high levels double your risk. High blood pressure also increases the chance of developing congestive heart failure and kidney disease. More than half of American women—and 70 percent of African American women—will develop high blood pressure at some point in their lives.

High blood pressure is called the "silent killer" because most people who have it do not feel sick. That means it is important to have your blood pressure checked regularly. Your doctor or other health professional should check your blood pressure on several different days before deciding whether it is too high. If your blood pressure stays at 140/90 millimeters of mercury (mmHg) or above, it is high and needs to be lowered.

What You Can Do: Control and Prevention

If you have high blood pressure, you can control it with proper treatment. If you don't have high blood pressure now, you can take steps to prevent it from developing. You can help to prevent and control high blood pressure by taking the following steps:

Limit your alcohol use. If you drink alcohol, have no more than one drink per day. That means no more than 12 ounces of beer, 5 ounces of wine, or 1 1/2 ounces of 80-proof liquor.

National Heart, Lung, and Blood Institute (NHLBI), NIH Publication No. 97-3655, revised September 1997.

Use less salt and sodium. Americans eat more salt (sodium chloride) and other forms of sodium than they need. And they also have higher rates of high blood pressure than people in other countries who eat less salt.

Women, and especially those with high blood pressure, should eat no more than about 6 grams of salt a day, which equals about 2,400 milligrams of sodium. That's about 1 teaspoon of table salt. This includes all salt eaten—including that in processed foods and added during cooking or at the table.

Be physically active. Moderate physical activity, if done regularly, can help control and prevent high blood pressure. Examples are brisk walking, gardening, yard work, housework, dancing, and home exercise. Try to do one or more of these activities for at least 30 minutes daily. The 30 minutes do not have to be done at one time, but can be broken into periods of at least 10 minutes each.

Lose weight if you are overweight. Taking off excess pounds will help to control and prevent high blood pressure, and will lower your chances of developing cardiovascular disease in several other ways. Weight loss will help to prevent and control diabetes, and it can also lower blood cholesterol levels. Finally, since overweight itself raises the chances of developing heart disease, losing weight can lower your risk.

Following are some suggestions for making weight loss an easier, safer, and more successful process:

- **Take it slowly.** The safest course is to take off weight gradually—no more than 1/2 pound to 1 pound per week. Don't think of weight control as a quick fix, but as a healthful, lifelong habit.

- **Eat for health.** Choose a wide variety of low-calorie, nutritious foods in moderate amounts from the basic food groups. Make sure that these foods are low in fat, since fat is the greatest source of calories. If you have a lot of weight to lose, ask your doctor, a registered dietitian, or a qualified nutritionist to help you develop a sensible, well-balanced plan for gradual weight loss

- **Keep milk on the menu.** Don't cut out dairy products in trying to reduce calories and fat. Dairy products are rich in calcium, a nutrient that is particularly important for women. Instead, choose non-fat or low fat dairy products.

- **Get beyond dieting.** To keep the pounds off, change your basic eating habits rather than simply "go on a diet." Learn to recognize social and emotional situations that trigger overeating and find ways to cope with them that work for you.

- **Avoid fads and diet pills.** Most fad diets provide poor nutrition and cause a number of side effects. Although fad diets can give quick and dramatic results, the weight returns quickly once you stop dieting. Also avoid diet pills. Most have troublesome side effects and none of them have been proven to work for long-term weight loss.

- **Get a move on.** Physical activity can help burn calories, tone muscles, maintain flexibility and good bone health, and control appetite. It will also help you keep off the weight you lose. Even moderate activity, such as brisk walking, will burn up calories and help control weight.

- **Ask for support.** Tell your family and friends about your weight loss plans and let them know how they can help you. You might also want to join a self-help group devoted to weight control. These groups provide support and practical suggestions on nutrition and long-term weight control.

If You Take Birth Control Pills

Although it is rare, it is important to know that if you take birth control pills, your blood pressure might increase. If you are taking oral contraceptives, you should get your blood pressure checked regularly. If you develop high blood pressure, you should ask your doctor about changing pills or stopping the pill and switching to another form of birth control.

Taking Blood Pressure Medication

If you have high blood pressure and it stays high even after you make the lifestyle changes described, your doctor will probably also prescribe medicine. The amount you take may be gradually reduced by your doctor, especially if you are successful with the changes you make in your lifestyle. If you feel any uncomfortable side effects from the drug, ask your doctor about lowering the amount you take, changing the type of medication, or adding another drug.

A reminder: It is very important to take a blood pressure medication exactly as your doctor has prescribed it. If you are not sure about your doctor's instructions, call to ask about the amount of medicine you are supposed to take each day, and the specific times of day you should be taking it.

Hold the Salt

How to Reduce Salt and Sodium in Your Diet

You can help prevent and control high blood pressure by cutting down on table salt and on sodium, an ingredient in salt that is found in many packaged foods. Following are some tips:

- If possible, reduce the amount a little each day until none is used. Try seasoning foods instead with pepper, garlic, ginger, minced onion or green pepper, and lemon juice.

- Use fewer sauces, mixes, and "instant" products, including flavored rices, pasta, and cereals, since they usually have salt added.

- Use fresh, frozen, or canned fruits.

- Use vegetables that are fresh, frozen without sauce, or canned with no salt added.

- Check nutrition labels for the amount of sodium in foods, especially on cans, boxes, bottles, and bags. Look for products that say "sodium free," "very low sodium," "low sodium," "reduced sodium," "less sodium," "light in sodium," or "unsalted."

- While salt substitutes containing potassium chloride may be useful for some individuals, they can be harmful to people with certain medical conditions. Ask your doctor before trying salt substitutes.

Congestive Heart Failure

An Important Reason to Control Your Blood Pressure

High blood pressure is the number one risk factor for congestive heart failure (CHF). Heart failure is a serious condition in which the heart is unable to pump enough blood to supply the body's needs. As a result, blood gets backed up in the veins, causing fluid to begin to seep into surrounding tissues. CHF causes excess fluid to accumulate in the lungs, producing breathing difficulties, fatigue and weakness, and sleeping problems.

In recent years, rates of hospitalization and death for CHF have been increasing in older Americans, especially women. One reason may be that many women do not adequately control their high blood pressure. Older women must be especially careful to continue taking blood pressure medication regularly—and also to take the right amount.

To reduce the risk of CHF, heart attack, and stroke, blood pressure should be controlled to 140/90 mmHg or lower. However, many women who are taking medication still have blood pressure that is

Table 13.1 Blood Pressure Categories in Women (18 Years and Older)*

Blood pressure is shown as two numbers—the systolic pressure as the heart is beating and the diastolic pressure between heartbeats. Both numbers are important.

	Blood Pressure Level in mmHg		
Category	*Systolic*		*Diastolic*
Optimal**	<120	and	<80
Normal	<130	and	<85
High-normal	130-139	or	85-89
Hypertension			
Stage 1	140-159	or	90-99
Stage 2	160-179	or	100-109
Stage 3	>180	or	>110

*Not taking antihypertensive drugs and not acutely ill. When systolic and diastolic blood pressures fall into different categories, the higher category determines blood pressure status.

**Optimal blood pressure with respect to cardiovascular risk is <120/ <80 mmHg. Unusually low readings should be evaluated for clinical significance.

Source: The Sixth Report of the Joint National Committee on Prevention, Detection, Evaluation, and Treatment of High Blood Pressure, NIH, NHLBI, 1997.

too high. There are various causes. Some women may not take their drugs as prescribed; for others, a drug may not lower blood pressure enough. If your blood pressure is higher than 140/90 mmHg, talk with your doctor about adjusting your medication and making lifestyle changes that will result in a blood pressure of 140/90 mmHg or lower.

What about Potassium?

Research shows that eating a lot of fruits and vegetables and non or low fat dairy products can lower blood pressure. Such foods supply plenty of potassium, magnesium, fiber, and calcium. Potassium, in particular, seems to prevent high blood pressure. Most women can get enough potassium in foods. Good sources of potassium are many fruits and vegetables, some dairy products, and fish.

Chapter 14

Be Physically Active

Physical Activity: Why Bother?

Physical inactivity increases the risk of heart disease. It both contributes directly to heart-related problems and increases the chances of developing other conditions that raise heart disease risk, such as high blood pressure and diabetes.

But the good news is that regular physical activity can help you reduce your risk of coronary heart disease, according to the first Surgeon General's Report on Physical Activity and Health as well as a National Institutes of Health expert panel. The reasons: Staying active helps take off extra pounds, helps to control blood pressure, boosts the level of "good" HDL-cholesterol, helps to prevent diabetes, and helps to prevent heart attacks.

For those who have heart disease, regular, moderate physical activity lowers the risk of death from heart-related causes. However, if you have heart disease, check with your doctor first to find out what kinds of activities are best for you.

Physical activity has many other benefits. It strengthens the lungs, tones the muscles, keeps the joints in good condition, improves balance, helps prevent and treat depression, and helps many people cope better with stress and anxiety.

National Heart, Lung, and Blood Institute (NHLBI), NIH Publication No. 97-3656, revised September 1997; with selected excerpts from *Heart Healthy Handbook for Women*, National Heart, Lung, and Blood Institute (NHLBI), NIH Publication No. 98-3654, revised August 1998.

Older women, in particular, can benefit from physical activities that strengthen bones and promote coordination and balance. Exercises such as T'ai Chi can improve balance and may be done alternately with heart-healthy physical activities. The National Institute on Aging (NIA) has a list of physical activities that are particularly helpful for older individuals. (For more information, write to the NIA Information Center at PO. Box 8057, Gaithersburg, MD 20898-8057; or phone 1-(800) 222-2225.)

What Kind of Activity Promotes Heart Health?

To reap benefits from physical activity, you don't need to train for a marathon. You need to engage in only about 30 minutes of moderate-level activity on most—and preferably all—days. A moderate-level activity is one that's about as demanding as brisk walking.

Other examples of everyday activities that can improve heart health are bicycling, housecleaning, raking leaves, and gardening. You can engage in any of these activities for 30 minutes at one time, or you can do them in shorter periods of at least 10 minutes each, as long as you total approximately 30 minutes per day. You also can do some of the 30 minutes in one activity and some in another.

If you are already engaging in this recommended level of physical activity, you will receive extra health and fitness benefits from doing these activities for a longer period each day, or by becoming involved in more vigorous activity.

Your Doctor Can Help

Some people should get medical advice before starting a program of physical activity. Consult your doctor before you begin or increase physical activity if you:

• Have heart trouble or have had a heart attack.

• Are taking medicine for high blood pressure or a heart condition.

• Are over 50 years old and are not used to moderately energetic activity.

• Have someone in your family who developed heart disease at an early age.

The Keys to Success

Go slow. If you have not been physically active until now, gradually build up to the recommended 30 minutes per day of moderate-level activity. For example, if you are inactive now and want to begin walking regularly, you might begin slowly with a 10-15 minute walk three times a week. As you become more fit, you can increase the sessions to every day. If you wish, you also can gradually lengthen each walking session or increase your pace.

Begin each workout slowly. Allow a 5-minute period of stretching and slow movement to give your body a chance to "warm up." At the end of your workout, take another 5 minutes to "cool down" with a slower pace.

Listen to your body. A certain amount of stiffness is normal at first. But if you hurt a joint or pull a muscle or tendon, stop the activity for several days to avoid more serious injury. Most minor muscle and joint problems can be relieved by rest and over-the-counter painkillers.

Pay attention to warning signals. While regular physical activity can strengthen your heart, some types of activity may worsen existing heart problems. Warning signals include sudden dizziness, cold sweat, paleness, fainting, or pain or pressure in your upper body or chest while—or just after—engaging in an activity. If you notice any of these signs, stop the activity and call your doctor immediately.

Check the weather report. On hot, humid days, do outdoor activities during the cooler and less humid parts of the day. Wear light, loose-fitting clothing and drink lots of water before, during, and after the activity. On cold days, wear one layer less of clothing than you would wear if you were outside but not physically active. Also wear gloves and a hat.

Keep at it. Unless you have to stop your regular physical activity for a health reason, stay with it. Set small, short-term goals for yourself. If you find yourself becoming bored, try doing the activity with a friend or family member. Or switch to another activity. The health rewards of regular physical activity are well worth the effort.

Making Opportunities

To become more physically active throughout your day, take advantage of any opportunity to get up and move around. For example:

- Use the stairs—up and down—instead of the elevator. Start with one flight of stairs and gradually build up to more.

- Park a few blocks front the office or store and walk the rest of the way. Or, if you ride on public transportation, get off a stop or two early and walk a few blocks.

- Instead of eating that extra snack, take a brisk stroll around the neighborhood.

- Do housework, such as vacuuming, at a brisker pace.

- Mow your own lawn.

- Carry your own groceries.

- Take an exercise break—get up and stretch, walk around and give your muscles and mind a chance to relax.

Table 14.1. Calories Burned Per Hour of Activity

Activity	Calories Burned Per Hour*
Bicycling, 6 mph	240
Bicycling, 12 mph	410
Cross-country skiing	700
Jogging, 5.5 mph	740
Jogging, 7 mph	920
Running in place	650
Swimming, 25 yds/min.	275
Swimming, 50 yds/min.	500
Tennis, singles	400
Walking, 2 mph	240
Walking, 3 mph	320
Walking, 4.5 mph	440

*For a healthy 150-pound woman. A lighter person burns fewer calories; a heavier person burns more.

Source: *Exercise and Your Heart*, National Heart, Lung, and Blood Institute, 1993.

Healthy Moves

Thirty minutes or more of moderate activity each day are good for your heart health. Here are some examples of moderate physical activities and chores that can reduce your risk of heart disease:

- Walking briskly (3-4 miles per hour)
- Conditioning or general calisthenics
- Housework
- Racquet sports, such as table tennis
- Lawn mowing (with power mower)
- Golf (pulling cart or carrying clubs)
- Home repair; house painting
- Jogging
- Swimming (moderate effort)
- Cycling, moderate speed (10 mph or less)
- Gardening
- Canoeing, leisurely pace (2-3.9 mph)
- Dancing

Source: *Dietary Guidelines for Americans*, U.S. Department of Agriculture/U.S. Department of Health and Human Services, 1995.

The Benefits of Regular Physical Activity

Regular activity can help you feel better because it:

- Boosts energy
- Helps you cope with stress
- Improves self-image
- Helps prevent fatigue
- Helps counter anxiety and depression
- Helps you relax and feel less tense
- Improves your ability to fall asleep and to sleep well
- Provides an easy way to share time with friends or family and to meet new friends

Regular activity can help you look better because it:

- Tones muscles
- Burns off calories to help you stay at your desirable weight, or to lose extra pounds
- Helps control your appetite

For More Information

If you want to know more about keeping your heart healthy, the National Heart, Lung, and Blood Institute (NHLBI) has available free fact sheets on the following subjects:

- preventing and controlling high blood pressure
- preventing and controlling high blood cholesterol
- quitting smoking
- heart disease risk factors for women

Contact:

NHLBI Information Center
P.O. Box 30105
Bethesda, MD 20824-0105
Phone: (301)251-1222
Fax: (301) 251-1223
Or check out the NHLBI web site at http://www.nhlbi.nih.gov/ nhlbi/ nhlbi.htm

Table 14.2. A Sample Walking Program

	Warm Up	Activity	Cool Down	Total Time
Week 1				
Session A	Walk slowly	Then walk briskly	Then walk slowly	
	5 min.	5 min.	5 min.	15 min.
Session B	Repeat above pattern			
Session C	Repeat above pattern			

Continue with at least three exercise sessions during each week of the program.

Table 14.2. A Sample Walking Program (continued)

Week 2

| Walk slowly 5 min. | Walk briskly 7 min. | Walk slowly 5 min. | 17 min. |

Week 3

| Walk slowly 5 min. | Walk briskly 9 min. | Walk slowly 5 min. | 19 min. |

Week 4

| Walk slowly 5 min. | Walk briskly 11 min. | Walk slowly 5 min. | 21 min. |

Week 5

| Walk slowly 5 min. | Walk briskly 13 min. | Walk slowly 5 min. | 23 min. |

Week 6

| Walk slowly 5 min. | Walk briskly 15 min. | Walk slowly 5 min. | 25 min. |

Week 7

| Walk slowly 5 min. | Walk briskly 18 min. | Walk slowly 5 min. | 28 min. |

Week 8

| Walk slowly 5 min. | Walk briskly 20 min. | Walk slowly 5 min. | 30 min. |

Week 9

| Walk slowly 5 min. | Walk briskly 23 min. | Walk slowly 5 min. | 33 min. |

Week 10

| Walk slowly 5 min. | Walk briskly 26 min. | Walk slowly 5 min. | 36 min. |

Week 11

| Walk slowly 5 min. | Walk briskly 28 min. | Walk slowly 5 min. | 38 min. |

Week 12 and Beyond

| Walk slowly 5 min. | Walk briskly 30 min. | Walk slowly 5 min. | 40 min. |

Chapter 15

A New Way to Think about Thighs

Not long ago Denise Arnold came across a photo of herself on a fishing trip she'd taken in junior high. In the picture she saw a blond teenager wearing snug knit shorts and a T-shirt, proudly holding up a 15-inch halibut. She also saw early signs of trouble. "You could already see the bumps coming," she says.

Now, more than 30 years later, Arnold will say good-bye to the bumps—the bulges of fat on her thighs. "I can't believe they're going to be gone," say the 47-year-old mother three from Las Vegas. "They're like old friends. They've been a part of me forever." She hesitates. "Well, I don't know if I'd call them friends. Friends you actually like."

Arnold dislikes her thighs so much that she is paying $10,000 to have the fat sucked out of them. After contemplating liposuction for years, she has decided to go through with it because of advances that have made the surgery safer, the recovery swifter, and the results more attractive.

But her timing is ironic. Just as cosmetic surgeons are making it easier for women to get rid of their thigh fat, researchers are offering them a compelling reason to hang on to it: "It turns out that the fat we so desperately want to get rid of might actually be good for us," says Glenn Gaesser, a University of Virginia exercise physiologist whose book *Big Fat Lies* argues that thinner is not necessarily

Health, January-February 1997, Vol. 11, No. 1, Pg. 44(3), © 1997 HEALTH; reprinted with permission.

healthier. In some cases, researchers speculate, removing thigh fat may even pose a long-term risk.

We've known for years that saddlebags are less harmful than a spare tire—that pear-shaped people are at lower risk for heart disease and diabetes than those shaped like apples. But now researchers suspect that "excess" thigh fat may pose no threat at all; in fact, for people who are also chunky around the middle, it may offer protection from disease.

Consider a study conducted at Stanford University. Scientists drew blood from 263 moderately overweight men and women, and evaluated factors that predict risk for heart disease: triglycerides (fats floating in the blood), LDL (the bad kind of cholesterol), and HDL (the good stuff). The subjects were then divided into three groups based on the size of their waists—small, medium, or large.

"Within each of the groups we found that the larger the thighs, the lower the risk," says the study's lead author Richard Terry, a research associate in Stanford's school of medicine. Other researchers agree: Extra thigh fat seems to counteract the risk from fat in the gut.

Scientists have some idea why. Most above-the-waist fat is stored deep in the belly, clumped around organs. These fat cells pose a problem because they're hubs of ceaseless activity from which fat molecules constantly come and go. And when these molecules are spit back into the bloodstream, in the form of fatty acids, they head straight to the liver, where they're repackaged with cholesterol and sent off to ravage the heart and arteries as triglycerides and LDL.

Thigh fat cells, on the other hand, sit just beneath the skin and operate at a much less frenetic pace; when fat molecules arrive in the thighs, they settle in and stay a long, long time. "Thigh fat takes the fat in the system out of circulation and keeps it safe," Terry says.

Denise Arnold knows just how stubborn thigh fat can be. For seven years she has walked an hour a day, even when she lived in Anchorage, Alaska, and the temperature would drop to ten degrees below zero. Determined to improve her health while slimming her thighs, Arnold also revamped her diet, filling her fridge with cut watermelon, cantaloupe, and nectarines. In the process she lost 30 pounds, but while her waist became trim, her bumps didn't budge.

Surgery isn't a decision Arnold came to hastily. She knows about the health benefits of being pear-shaped and about the potential complications of liposuction—infection, nerve damage, brown spots and dents in the skin, adverse reactions to anesthesia, and excessive fluid loss that can lead to shock. But she's tired of being embarrassed by her thighs.

"I'm not doing this so I can prance up and down the beach," she says. "I just want to be able to wear jeans without having to wear panty hose and a girdle underneath."

Complications from liposuction are rare. But what about the risks after surgery? Could the loss of a couple billion fat cells compromise a woman's long-term health? In some cases, researchers think, a woman who gains weight after surgery may have cause for worry. "If a woman has a lot of thigh fat taken out and she doesn't have a lot of fat to begin with, she might be looking at a metabolic time bomb," Gaesser says. In other words, if the body routes enough fat to the abdomen because it has nowhere else to put it, a liposuction patient's risk for heart disease might rise.

Gaesser is speculating, because no one has followed up on liposuction patients years after surgery. Three plastic surgeons ran a short study, comparing the blood fat of 30 patients before surgery and three months after. "We found no change," says Joseph Hunstad, the North Carolina surgeon who led the study.

The work of New York surgeon John Kral, however, suggests that removing large amounts of thigh fat might be a bad idea. Kral performed lipectomies (cutting away fat rather than sucking it out) on two obese women, taking more than ten pounds of fat from each. Within six months both women had slightly raised triglyceride levels and performed poorly on a glucose tolerance test, indicating a greater risk for diabetes. These findings imply that their abdominal fat may have grown after surgery, a theory supported by animal studies. When rats have fat removed from beneath the skin, the amount stored in their abdominal area increases.

But researchers say Denise Arnold has nothing to worry about. She won't be losing more than a few pounds of fat-not enough, they agree, to alter her blood fat profile. And her salutary eating and exercise habits should protect her heart.

As Arnold lies half naked on the operating table, the rewards of her lifestyle are obvious. Her stomach is flat, her arms are trim, her calves are sculpted. "She's the ideal candidate for liposuction because she has a distortion in her figure, not a weight problem," says Alan Gaynor, her surgeon, who practices in San Francisco. A former liposuction recipient himself, he is eager to rid his patient of her "guitar shape."

Numb from the chest down, Arnold is undergoing "tumescent" liposuction: Her thighs have been injected with a solution that causes the fat cells to swell (that is, to become tumescent) and the blood vessels to constrict; it also serves as an anesthetic.

This technique, now used by most cosmetic surgeons, has made liposuction less traumatic. Patients bleed much less, so doctors are able to safely remove as much as seven pounds of fat—four times more than when the solution isn't used. (The latest technique, ultrasonic liposuction, which is now being tested at half a dozen surgery centers around the country, will allow doctors to remove even more fat.) And though patients may still feel pain and soreness for a day or two after surgery, they have significantly less bruising. Typically they're able to walk comfortably in a few days and ease back into their exercise routines m a couple of weeks.

Arnold's surgery is a three-part process. To suck out the deeper thigh fat, Gaynor attaches the hose of a powerful vacuum to a foot-long cannula—a flexible tube connected to a blunt metal rod with a hole near the tip. He slips the device into one thigh through a small incision, then thrusts it back and forth, like a fencer making quick jabs. Inside the cannula, yellow chunks of fat blend with a little blood, forming a thick, orange goo that spirals down into a canister that looks like the pitcher of a blender.

Later, with both thighs slimmed down and the canister almost full, Gaynor starts the fine-tuning. He discards the vacuum hose and attaches a narrower cannula to a large syringe; when he pulls the plunger out, the fat gets suctioned up. This method allows surgeons to extract fat with more precision than in the past, when only large cannulas and vacuums were used; as a result, skin ends up with technique "liposculpting."

When he has finished removing all of the fat he deems necessary, Gaynor uses an even smaller rod to scratch just underneath Arnold's skin. The scratching causes tiny grooves in the tissue, he says. When these heal in the months following surgery, Arnold's skin will contract, lessening unsightly sagging.

No one knows what percent of liposuction patients keep off the fat. One study of nine patients found that four gained most of it back within a year. But cosmetic surgeons maintain that liposuction is permanent as long as you exercise regularly and eat sensibly.

Even if you did gain back fat, they say, your thighs wouldn't get a disproportionate amount because you have lost billions of fat cells; your remaining fat cells, now more evenly distributed, would simply get larger (a result that may make patients happy, but concerns researchers like Terry). However, this question has never been formally studied in liposuction patients.

Research does show that new fat cells can actually appear in pregnant women and in people who gain massive amounts of weight. But nobody knows whether fat cells might reappear in the thighs of a patient such as Denise Arnold.

Arnold, for one, has no intention of finding out. Three weeks after surgery she is already forgetting the immediate postsurgical pain ("as bad as natural childbirth") and is so inspired by the results that she's upped her daily walk to over an hour.

"I was in Macy's the other day, and the swimsuits were 75 percent off," says Arnold. "Just for fun I tried one on, and I couldn't believe the back view. I just stood there and stared in the mirror. All my life I've been self-conscious about my bumps. And now they're gone."

— by Suzanne Schlosberg

Chapter 16

Kicking the Smoking Habit

Cigarette smoking is a habit that greatly increases your chances of developing cardiovascular diseases. Surprising as it may seem, smoking by women in this country causes 1.5 times the number of deaths from heart disease and stroke as from lung cancer. If you smoke, you are two to six times more likely to suffer a heart attack than a nonsmoking woman, and the risk increases with the number of cigarettes you smoke each day. Smoking also increases the risk of stroke.

Smoking also poses many other health risks for women. For instance, women who smoke lose bone mass more quickly after menopause than those who do not smoke. And cigarette smoke doesn't just put your health at risk, it also affects those around you, including children.

In short, there is simply no safe way to smoke. Although low-tar and low-nicotine cigarettes may reduce the lung cancer risk somewhat, they do not lessen the risks of heart diseases. The only safe and healthful course is not to smoke at all.

If you now use cigarettes, you can stop. There are as many ex-smokers in this country today as there are smokers. Becoming a successful ex-smoker is what this chapter is all about.

The Good News about Quitting

There is nothing easy about giving up cigarettes. But as hard as quitting may be, the results are well worth it. One year after you stop

National Heart, Lung, and Blood Institute (NHLBI), NIH Publication No. 97-3657, revised September 1997.

smoking, your risk of coronary heart disease will drop by more than half. Within several years, it will approach the heart disease risk of someone who never smoked.

This means that no matter what your age, quitting will lessen your chances of developing heart disease.

Meanwhile, for those who now have heart disease, giving up cigarettes lowers the risk of a heart attack. Quitting also reduces the risk of a second heart attack in women who have already had one.

Take some time to think about other benefits of being an ex-smoker. Note the reasons that apply to you in the section below, "Why I Want to Quit Smoking." Consider other reasons you think are important. This is an important first step in kicking the smoking habit figuring out for yourself what you have to gain.

Why I Want to Quit Smoking

- I will greatly lessen my chances of having a heart attack or stroke.
- I will greatly lessen my chances of getting lung cancer, emphysema, and other lung diseases.
- I will have fewer colds or flu each year.
- I will have better smelling clothes, hair, breath, home, and car.
- I will climb stairs and walk without getting out of breath.
- I will have fewer wrinkles.
- I will be free of my morning cough.
- I will reduce the number of coughs, colds, and earaches my children have.
- I will have more energy to pursue physical activities.
- I will have more control over my life.
- I will.......

Getting Ready to Quit

Once you decide to stop smoking, you'll need to set a target date for quitting. Choose a time when you won't be under a lot of stress. To help you stick to your quit date, write "I will quit smoking on (fill in the date)" on a piece of paper and have someone sign it with you. Now you have a contract. Also, list on your contract how you'll reward yourself for each week and month of not smoking.

Ask the person who co-signs your contract—or another friend or family member—to give you special support in your efforts to quit. Plan to talk with your supporter regularly to share your progress and to ask for encouragement. If possible, quit with a relative or friend.

Breaking the Habit

Surviving "Day One." On the evening before your quit day, throw away all cigarettes, matches, lighters, and ashtrays. Plan some special activities for the next day to keep you busy, such as a long walk, a movie, or an outing with a friend. Ask family members and friends not to offer you cigarettes or to smoke in front of you. Your goal is to get through that first important day smoke-free—which will help you succeed on each day after that.

Know Yourself. To quit successfully, you need to know your smoking "triggers," which are situations and feelings that bring on the urge to light up. Common triggers are drinking coffee, finishing a meal, watching television, having an alcoholic drink, talking on the phone, watching someone else smoke, or being under stress. Make a list of your personal smoking triggers and avoid as many as you can.

Find New Habits. Replace "triggers" with new activities that you don't associate with smoking. For example, if you always had a cigarette with a cup of coffee, switch to tea for a while. If you're feeling tense, try deep breathing to calm yourself. (Take a slow, deep breath, count to five, and release it. Repeat 10 times.)

Keep Busy. Get involved in projects that require you to use your hands, such as sewing or jigsaw puzzles. When you feel the urge to put something in your mouth, have low calorie substitutes ready, such as vegetable sticks, apple slices, or sugarless gum.

Be Physically Active. Walk, garden, or bicycle. Physical activity will make you feel better and help prevent weight gain.

Know What to Expect. Shortly after quitting, you may experience headaches, irritability, tiredness, constipation, or trouble concentrating. While these symptoms are not pleasant, it is important to know that they are signs that your body is recovering from smoking. Most symptoms end within 2 to 4 weeks.

Help Is Available. There are many free or low-cost programs available to help you stop smoking. Check with local chapters of the American Lung Association and the American Cancer Society, area hospitals, health maintenance organizations (HMOs), your workplace, and community groups with an interest in health.

Be Good to Yourself. Get plenty of rest, drink lots of fluids, and eat three balanced, healthful meals each day. If you are not as cheerful or energetic as usual during the first several weeks after quitting, don't feel guilty. You are making a major change in your life, and for that you deserve a lot of credit.

If You "Slip"

A slip means that you have had a small setback and smoked a cigarette after your quit date. Don't worry. Most smokers slip three to five times before they quit for good. But to get right back on the nonsmoking track, here are some tips:

- *Don't Get Discouraged.* Having a cigarette or two doesn't mean you have failed. It doesn't mean you can't quit smoking. Keep thinking of yourself as a nonsmoker. You are one.

- *Learn From Experience.* What was the trigger that made you light up? Were you having a drink at a party or feeling angry at someone? Think back on the day's events until you can remember.

- *Take Charge.* Make a list of things you will do the next time you are in that situation—and other tempting situations as well. Reread your list of all the reasons you want to quit. You're on your way.

A Weighty Concern

Many women fear that if they stop smoking they will gain unwanted weight. But most ex-smokers gain less than 10 pounds. Weight gain may be partly due to changes in the way the body uses calories after smoking stops. Also, some people eat more when quitting because they substitute high-calorie foods for cigarettes. Choosing more lower-calorie foods and boosting your physical activity level can reduce weight gain.

If you do gain some weight, you can work on losing it after you have become comfortable as a nonsmoker. When you think about the enormous health risks of smoking, the possibility of putting on a few pounds is not a reason to continue.

Three Aids for Quitting

As you prepare to quit smoking, give serious consideration to using a nicotine aid to help you stay off cigarettes. Three products—nicotine gum, a nicotine patch, and a nicotine nasal spray—can help you successfully quit by lessening your withdrawal symptoms. The gum and patch are now available over-the-counter, while the nasal spray is available only by prescription.

However, nicotine aids are not for everyone. Pregnant women, nursing mothers, and people with serious heart problems cannot use them safely. Talk with your doctor about whether you should try any of these aids.

Stopping Smoking's Triggers

You probably have certain situations and feelings that trigger your desire to smoke. Do you smoke while on the telephone? After having a meal or a drink? When you feel stressed?

To make stopping easier, find out what your triggers are—and then come up with alternate behaviors. Have a slice of apple or a stick of sugar-free gum, for instance, rather than a cigarette.

Chapter 17

How Passive Is Passive Smoking?

"Passive smoking," or environmental tobacco smoke (ETS), has significant health consequences for nonsmokers. Exposure to cigarette smoke at home or at work increases a nonsmoker's risk of coronary artery disease by up to 30%. And each year between 37,000 and 40,000 nonsmokers die of cardiovascular disease caused by cigarette smoke. These sobering statistics have launched many legislative efforts to ban smoking in public places. And two recent studies add weight to those arguments.

Passive Smoking and Heart Disease

Data from the Nurses' Health Study document that regular exposure to cigarette smoke at home or at work nearly doubles a woman's risk of heart disease. Researchers—including Harvard Heart Letter editorial board members Walter C. Willett, MD, and Charles H. Hennekens, MD—focused on 32,046 women who were 36-61 years old in 1982. At that time, all of these women reported that they had never smoked, and all were free of known coronary artery disease, stroke, or cancer.

Although all the women were nonsmokers, about 80% of them reported regular or occasional exposure to environmental tobacco smoke at home or work. More than 10,000 of the women reported regular exposure. During the next 10 years, 25 of these women died from coronary

Excerpted from May, 1998 issue of *Harvard Heart Letter*, © 1998 President and Fellows of Harvard College; reprinted with permission.

artery disease and another 127 had nonfatal heart attacks. After adjusting for other heart-attack risk factors, researchers found that women reporting regular exposure to cigarette smoke had a 91% increase in the risk of heart disease. Those who reported occasional exposure had a 58% increase in risk. While either workplace or home exposure was associated with an increase in heart-disease risk, that risk was greatly increased for women exposed to cigarette smoke both at home and at work.

In short, regular exposure to passive smoking at work or home increased the risk of coronary artery disease among nonsmoking women—a group generally considered at low risk for heart attack. This study illustrates that environmental tobacco smoke is a significant risk factor for heart disease. (*Circulation*, Vol. 95, No. 10, pp. 2374-2379.)

Cigarette Smoke and Atherosclerosis

The ARIC (Atherosclerosis Risk in Communities) study examined the effects of both "active" and passive smoking on blood vessels in 16,000 people, and the news is disturbing. To assess the effects of cigarette smoke on the progression of atherosclerosis, researchers used ultrasound to measure the thickness of the carotid arteries (the arteries in the neck that carry blood to the brain). This measurement was used to track the progression of atherosclerosis over three years in five groups:

- smokers
- past smokers who were regularly exposed to environmental tobacco smoke (ETS)
- past smokers who had not been exposed to ETS
- people who had never smoked but were exposed to ETS
- never-smokers who did not report ETS exposure

Over the study period, atherosclerosis progressed 50% in current smokers and 25% in past smokers. Compared to those not exposed to ETS, atherosclerosis increased by 20% in those with ETS exposure. That's roughly 34% of the rate for active smokers. And the detrimental effects of smoking proved much worse for people with diabetes or high blood pressure.

Does how much a person smokes influence the progression of atherosclerosis? Researchers also found that the greater the number of cigarettes smoked per day over time, the faster atherosclerosis progressed. But when comparing people who had smoked the same number of cigarettes, it didn't matter whether the study participants were current or past smokers; atherosclerosis progressed at the same rate in both groups. And atherosclerosis progressed 24% faster in former smokers than in never-smokers, implying that some of the smoking's effects on blood vessels may be irreversible. (*Journal of the American Medical Association*, Vol. 279, No. 2, pp. 119-124).

Clearing the Smoke

Data from these studies emphasize the dangers of environmental tobacco smoke and will inform the debate that surrounds banning smoking in public places. The suggestion that some of the effects of passive smoking may be permanent does not mean smokers shouldn't bother kicking the habit. Epidemiological studies continue to show that mortality rates from cardiovascular disease for former smokers return to that of never-smokers within three to five years of quitting. Simply put, cigarette smoke contributes to heart disease and other illnesses in a number of ways, and quitting reduces the risk. If anything, these studies should provide people with another good reason never to start.

Chapter 18

Aspirin as Prevention

The research on aspirin is promising: This well-known "wonder drug" may help to both prevent and treat heart attacks.

A study of more than 87,000 women found that those who took a low dose of aspirin regularly were less likely to suffer a first heart attack than women who took no aspirin. Women over age 50 appeared to benefit most. While earlier research has shown that aspirin can help prevent heart attacks in men, this was the first study to suggest a similar result for women.

Other recent research suggests that only a tiny daily dose of aspirin may be needed to protect against heart attacks. One study found that for both women and men, taking only 30 mg of aspirin daily— one-tenth the strength of a regular aspirin—helped prevent heart attacks as effectively as the usual 300 mg dose. The smaller dose also caused less stomach irritation.

Aspirin also reduces the chances that women who have already had a heart attack or stroke will have, or die from, another one. Aspirin may also increase the chances of survival after a heart attack, if it is taken quickly. A major study showed that taking a low dose of aspirin within the first hours of an attack reduced deaths by 23 percent.

However, you should not take aspirin either to treat or prevent a heart attack without first discussing it with your doctor. Aspirin is a powerful drug with many side effects. It can increase your chances of

Exerpted from *Heart Healthy Handbook for Women*, National Heart, Lung, and Blood Institute (NHLBI), NIH Publication No. 98-3654, revised August 1998.

getting ulcers, kidney disease, liver disease, and stroke from a hemorrhage. Only a doctor who knows your complete medical history and current health can judge whether the benefits you may gain from aspirin outweigh the risks.

Chapter 19

Advice for Staying Well during Life's Second Half

Over the next 5 years, 6 million American women will enter the age of menopause, swelling the ranks in that segment of the population to 54 million. In the 5 years after that, 6 million more will make the transition. What many are not aware of is that certain lifestyle habits can make a big difference in a menopausal or postmenopausal woman's health and well-being, in many cases even more of a difference than when she was in her childbearing years. The lack of awareness is to be expected. Researchers are only now putting the spotlight on women—specifically women in their late 40s and beyond—to pinpoint exactly what they need to do to remain healthy throughout the second half of their lives. The good news is that answers about how women should eat and otherwise take care of themselves are finally starting to come in. Here are 7 points of advice, some of them based on research findings that have been published only within the last several weeks.

1. Be aggressive about keeping down blood cholesterol.

Only 9 percent of postmenopausal women with heart disease have their "bad" LDL—cholesterol sufficiently under control, according to a newly released study of more than 2,700 postmenopausal women.

"The 7 Habits of Highly Health-Oriented Postmenopausal Women: Advice for Staying Well during Life's Second Half," in *Tufts University Health & Nutrition Letter*, June 1997, Vol. 15, No. 4, Pg. 4(2), © 1997; reprinted with permission, *Tufts University Health & Nutrition Letter*, Tel: 1-800-274-7581.

Almost half of the women were taking cholesterol-lowering medication, but apparently many of them were not getting prescriptions for the proper doses—or were not aware of how important it was for them to take their medicine as prescribed.

That's probably at least part of the reason why even in the group on medication, the average LDL—cholesterol concentration was up to 138 (milligrams per tenth of a liter of blood). The LDL-cholesterol level for a woman with heart disease is supposed to be below 100. Even for a woman without heart disease, the target is less than 130—lower than what the drug-taking women achieved.

The lower the LDL-cholesterol level, previous research has indicated, the slower the buildup of plaque that clogs arteries and the fewer heart attacks and other coronary problems. Lower cholesterol can be achieved not just by taking drugs but also by eating less saturated fat and losing excess weight.

Why the lack of sufficient treatment of women's cholesterol levels? First, there is the common misperception—among both physicians and many women themselves—that women are at a lower risk of dying from heart disease than men. Nothing could be further from the truth. Coronary heart disease is the leading cause of death among both men and women, particularly among women who have reached menopause. In fact, a 60-year-old woman is much more likely to die of heart disease than of breast cancer.

It is also erroneously thought in some circles that interventions such as lowering LDL levels to reduce heart disease risk are inherently less effective in women than in men. But women treated for high cholesterol appear to benefit as much as men do, if not more. In one study, women taking medication for moderately high blood cholesterol had a 46 percent reduction in coronary events, while men receiving the same drug experienced only a 20 percent reduction.

Bottom line: Do not take high blood cholesterol lightly, and do not let your physician take it lightly either.

2. Live longer by keeping active.

A study of more than 40,000 postmenopausal women published at the same time as the cholesterol study found that those who exercise outlive their sedentary counterparts. The higher their level of physical activity, the longer they live.

Even women who engaged just once a week in moderate physical activity such as golf, gardening, or taking a long walk were 20 to 25 percent less likely to die over a 7-year period than inactive women. Those who participated in moderate physical activity more than 4 times a week were about 40 percent less likely to die than their sedentary counterparts. Exercising regularly proved particularly effective at reducing the risk of respiratory and cardiovascular diseases.

Bottom line: At a minimum, take a long walk once a week. The more you exercise your body, the better.

3. Work to avoid putting on excess weight.

Many women believe that putting on pounds is a de facto part of menopause. Some on estrogen replacement therapy have voiced concern that it's the hormone that's causing them to gain weight. But weight gain is not generally a sign of menopause or menopause treatment but simply something that often accompanies aging.

Consider that basal metabolic rate—the rate at which the body expends calories while at rest for activities like breathing and cell maintenance—tends to drop an estimated 2 percent every decade starting at age 20. The result is that every 10 years, a person needs fewer calories a day to remain at the same weight.

Thus, if someone reaches her 50s eating the same amount she did in her 20s but not increasing her activity level to burn calories, she is bound to gain some weight. The more weight gained, the higher the risk for conditions often associated with later life, including diabetes and high blood pressure.

One way around the calorie-burning slowdown is to eat fewer calories. But another way for women to have their cake and at least eat some of it too is to engage twice a week in weight lifting and other strength-training activities.

Part of the reason calorie requirements decrease throughout adult life is that the body loses muscle, or lean mass, which is metabolically active tissue that requires calories to sustain itself. The rate of muscle loss accelerates after age 45. But strength-training exercises maintain and build muscle (and improve bone mass, as do aerobic activities). The more calories burned maintaining that muscle, the fewer stored in the body's fat cells.

Bottom line: Along with engaging in aerobic activities like brisk walking, maintain desirable weight by strength training 2 times a week. And "spend" calories wisely on nutrient-rich vegetables, fruits, dairy foods, and lean meats so you can enjoy the occasional (or even daily, in small amounts) chocolate or ice cream.

4. Get more calcium.

In part because of following diets that contain too little calcium, 1 out of 3 women over 50 will suffer a vertebral fracture, which can lead not only to stooped posture but also to severe back pain and difficulty breathing due to changes in the skeletal configuration. Thinning hones also cause more than 300,000 hip fractures a year, creating a risk that's equal to the risk of breast uterine and ovarian cancer combined. Here's the amount of calcium the National Institutes of Health (NIH) recommends for menopausal women to help prevent bone breaks:

- for women on estrogen replacement therapy under age 65: 1,000 milligrams a day

- for women not on estrogen replacement therapy under age 65: 1,500 milligrams a day

- for all women 65 and older: 1,500 milligrams a day

If those numbers seem high, it's because they are. On the other hand, a woman who makes a concerted effort to eat a truly balanced diet should be able to get close to 1,000 milligrams of calcium from foods. A cup of milk, which is not even enough to quite fill a tea cup to the rim, contains 300 milligrams. A cup of calcium-fortified orange juice contains at least 200 milligrams, as does an ounce of hard cheese. Smaller amounts of calcium can be found in vegetables, fruits, and beans. Thus, a menopausal woman who eats an overall good diet will need, at most, only about 500 to 600 milligrams of supplemental calcium daily.

Note: The body can't absorb enough calcium without enough vitamin D. And calcium is coming to light that postmenopausal women need more vitamin D than others—between 400 and 800 International Units a day, or 2 to 4 times the Recommended Dietary Allowance. Women who live in southern climes need not be too concerned, since their skin manufactures vitamin D upon exposure to sunlight. That's true even if they leave only small areas of their skin without sunscreen for just 10 to 15 minutes a day. But women who live in northern areas may want to take a multivitamin/mineral pill that contains 400 units of vitamin D, at least during the winter months. The nutrient is found in appreciable amounts in very few foods, including milk (100 units a cup), fatty fish, organ meats like liver, egg yolks, and fortified cereals (check the Nutrition Facts panel on the side of the box).

Bottom line: Work more dairy foods into a diet rounded out with fruits and vegetables. And don't forget the vitamin D factor. (But don't overdo. More than 1,000 units of D daily, can be toxic.)

5. Try soy.

You've probably heard that the phytoestrogens, or plant estrogens, in soy protein might help ease night sweats, mood swings, and other discomforts of menopause, not to mention play a role in keeping down blood cholesterol levels. But there's more.

Researchers are now coming upon some preliminary evidence that estrogens in soy foods may help prevent bone loss by inhibiting bone resorption—the process by which calcium is pulled from the bones and into the bloodstream. Some have suggested that such evidence may help explain why in Asian countries, where soy products are a much bigger part of the diet but high-calcium dairy foods are largely absent, there are not reports of rampant osteoporosis. In one study at the University of Illinois, postmenopausal women who ate a diet relatively rich in soy phytoestrogens known as isoflavones had an increase in bone mineral density in their spines, compared with women who ate little or no isoflavones. A study in Australia produced similar results. Scientists at the Monash Medical Center there found that feeding soy products to postmenopausal women for 12 weeks caused bone mineral density to increase.

Bottom line: Experiment with some soy-based foods. It doesn't have to be tofu. For instance, soy protein is often an ingredient in vegetarian chili. It can also be purchased in health food stores as soy protein isolate powder and sprinkled into smoothies and other concoctions made in the blender. And it comes in textured vegetable protein flakes that can be added to marinara sauce for body.

6. Get more folate.

Studies show that the B vitamin folate may help protect against heart disease. With an adequate amount of that nutrient in the diet, the blood contains less of a substance called homocysteine—a marker for heart disease risk similar to the way cholesterol is. Researchers believe that it would take 400 micrograms of folate a day to keep homocysteine levels low enough. Only 12 percent of Americans eat that much of the vitamin. Most eat more on the order of 200 micrograms.

133

Bottom line: Make sure to eat a well-rounded diet that has plenty of folate-rich foods, including chickpeas, lentils, and other legumes; orange juice; and green vegetables such as spinach.

7. Fight against depression.

Up to 2 out of 5 older Americans suffer from depression, which could blunt appetite—or at least make a woman pay less attention to eating a healthful diet than she should. Signs of depression include preferring to stay at home rather than go out and do the things you have always enjoyed; lacking energy; and feeling hopeless (although you should always speak to a health care provider rather than self-diagnose or treat yourself).

Bottom line: Don't accept the blues as an inevitable part of aging. Even people who lose a spouse do not have to spend the rest of their lives depressed, especially if they seek help and get proper social support. Exercise alone helps lift people's moods. Tufts researchers have found that depressed women with an average age of 70 who started strength training experienced a significant upturn in their outlook after just a couple of months.

Part Three

Treatment and Control Strategies

Chapter 20

Treating Heart Disease in Women

Heart disease is the leading cause of death among women over 40, causing more deaths annually than all forms of cancer combined. Underlying this, women have a tendency to develop heart disease later in life than men.

"Women tend to be treated for heart disease later than men," says Connie P. Anggelis, M.D., member of the Alliant adult medical staff, which serves Norton Hospital and Alliant Medical Pavilion. "At the time of treatment, their angina has generally progressed to a greater point and if it's progressed to a greater point, then the blockage is more significant and the risk goes up."

Angina is pain resulting from an ongoing lack of blood flow to the heart (ischemia) due to coronary artery disease. As the disease progresses, cholesterol-like material forms in the inner layer of the arteries, interfering with normal blood flow.

According to Anggelis, one key to successfully treating heart disease is to recognize the disease early. Risk factors, heredity and lifestyle all play a part.

"People don't recognize the signs of angina," says Anggelis. "When you say chest pain, people tend to think sharp but that's not what it is. It's a sort of crushing pain."

"Treating Heart Disease in Women," Information provided by the Norton Hospital Women's Pavilion Heart Center, © Norton Hospital, undated; reprinted with permission.

"If your discomfort is not relieved within five minutes you need to call your family physician or go to the emergency room. What you don't do is stay home and try to figure it out yourself."

"As a clinician, the first thing we do is try to make a diagnosis to see if a patient has coronary disease or not," says Janet Smith, M.D., also a member of the Alliant adult medical staff. "If she does have the disease, we try to get an idea of her risk for a heart attack. This is very important because patients who have coronary disease can sometimes have far fewer symptoms than you would expect for the extent of the disease."

Smith says risk category is often diagnosed from a combination of symptoms and exercise or stress testing.

"We know a patient is in a very high risk category if she comes in with pain that is classic for heart pain and a very unstable electrocardiogram. (An electrocardiogram is a test which measures electrical impulses from the heart.) We don't need to run a stress test to recognize that this patient is a high-risk patient." It is from this point that treatment can be determined.

According to Anggelis and Smith there are a number of medications available to treat heart disease.

"If we have diagnosed a blockage," says Anggelis, "and a stable pattern of pain is occurring, meaning that pain does not occur at rest or with increasing frequency over the last month, we can treat the patient with medication."

"Nitrates work to relieve pain by changing blood flow to the area of heart muscle. Some nitrates are used for episodic pain or can he used on a daily basis to decrease the chances of heart attack."

"Beta blockers are another type of drug used to treat heart disease. Beta blockers work by decreasing the heart rate and blood pressure. While they do decrease the demand on the heart for blood flow, beta blockers can have side effects on other systems of the body and are therefore used with caution."

"Calcium antagonists also can be prescribed. They not only decrease demand but also relax blood vessels and may dilate the arteries by slightly decreasing blood pressure and sometimes heart rate."

"If further treatment is needed, because of lack of pain control or an unstable pain pattern, anatomy will help us decide between surgery and catheter procedures," says Smith of the next line of defense to treat heart disease.

"Interventional procedures are done with a catheter. We go through the groin or the arm to deal with the artery. We may use a balloon, lasers, Rotablator®, which allow us to actually scrape out plaque, or stents that support the artery wall."

"All blockages are somewhat different. Some blockages are nice and soft, some are on a bend, some are hard and have calcium in them. The tool that we use is determined by the blockage," says Smith.

But Smith cautions, "Like medication, catheter procedures, as well as bypass surgery, are treatments for heart disease. They are not a cure. The problem with all catheter-based interventions is that there is a certain percentage of recurrence."

According to Smith, there is between a 30-percent and 50-percent chance of recurrence. If the blockage does recur, it will usually return during the first six- to 12-week period after the procedure. If the patient can get to the one-year mark without a recurrence, it is unlikely that particular artery will block again. However, heart disease is seldom in only one artery and other arteries and vessels are still vulnerable.

"Usually symptoms will be similar if there is a recurrence," says Smith. "The pain will come back or there will be a change in follow-up tests."

"Another thing to consider," says Smith, "is that there is a 3-percent to 5-percent chance of having to undergo emergency bypass surgery during a catheter procedure."

"The need for bypass surgery instead of a catheter procedure," Smith says, "is basically an anatomical decision and is typical for patients who have fairly extensive disease as well as those who have undergone several catheter procedures."

"In extreme cases, heart transplants are used."

"You would consider a transplant when either there has been so much muscle damage that the muscle itself is very weak or when the blockage is so far down in the vessels that there is really no good place to use a catheter or bypass," says Smith.

If heart disease symptoms are recognized early and treated immediately, the chance of surviving heart disease is good.

"Angina leads directly to the path of heart attack," emphasizes Anggelis, "The rule is to determine early on what kind of pain you're dealing with."

Chapter 21

So, You Have Heart Disease?

If you're a woman who has or thinks she has coronary heart disease, this chapter is for you. It explains the causes, symptoms, detection, and treatments of coronary heart disease.

Coronary heart disease is a chronic condition—it will not disappear—and you may need to make some changes. But caring for your heart is worth the effort—your heart will thank you every day.

A Long Process

Coronary heart disease, the most common form of heart disease, develops over many years. It can begin as far back as childhood. In a process known as atherosclerosis, fatty substances build up inside the walls of blood vessels. Blood components also stick on the surface inside vessel walls. The vessels narrow and "harden," becoming less flexible.

The buildup and narrowing proceed gradually and result in decreasing blood flow and, eventually, the development of symptoms. But the buildup, or "plaque," may break open and suddenly produce a blood clot, limited blood flow, and symptoms.

When blood flow to the heart is reduced, chest pain, or "angina," can result. If blood flow is nearly or completely blocked, a heart attack can occur and cause muscle cells in the heart to die. Because the cells cannot be replaced, the result is permanent heart damage.

National Heart, Lung, and Blood Institute (NHLBI), NIH Publication No. 96-2645, September 1996.

141

Who Gets Coronary Heart Disease?

Coronary heart disease rarely affects young women. Instead, it usually develops after menopause. Before menopause, the ovaries make estrogen, which helps protect the heart.

Being over age 55 is a "risk factor" that affects the development of coronary heart disease. There are other risk factors. They are: family history of early heart disease, cigarette smoking, high blood pressure, high blood cholesterol, being overweight, physical inactivity, and diabetes.

The risk factors do not add their effects in a simple way. Rather, they multiply each other's effects. For example, if you smoke and have high blood pressure and high blood cholesterol, you're eight times more likely to develop coronary heart disease than a woman with no risk factors.

You can have coronary heart disease without being aware of it. The best way to protect your heart is to know whether you have coronary heart disease and treat it as early as possible. You need to talk to your doctor about your coronary heart disease and any symptoms you may be experiencing.

Do You Have Angina?

The first symptom of coronary heart disease may be chest pain, or "angina." The chest pain, which is caused by reduced blood flow to the heart, typically occurs behind the breastbone and may travel down your left arm or up your neck, or be a squeezing, pressing sensation that does not change with breathing. It is usually caused and made worse by exercise and eased by rest. The pain usually lasts 2 to 5 minutes. If you have this kind of chest pain, you should contact your doctor.

A reduced blood flow to the heart can cause symptoms other than chest pain. For example, some women get a less typical angina. The chest pain may linger, occur in a different location than behind the breastbone, or not be worsened by exertion and eased by rest. Some women have shortness of breath or indigestion. If you have such symptoms, you should talk with your doctor. If treated, the outlook is good. Without treatment, however, the symptoms may recur and worsen and can become unstable and even lead to a heart attack.

Women who have coronary heart disease need to talk to their doctor about the symptoms of a heart attack and the appropriate steps to take to get emergency care. It is important to know the telephone number to call to get emergency transportation to the hospital. In most areas, this will be 9-1-1 or a 7-digit emergency number.

Getting to the hospital fast allows use of thrombolytic therapy—a clot-dissolving agent is injected to restore blood flow through an artery. This therapy saves lives and reduces damage to the heart muscle. But it must be done as soon as possible.

Doctors also have a new fast test for a heart attack. It detects changed levels of an enzyme (creatine kinase MB) produced by the heart. It once took up to a day to test the levels and tell if someone has had a heart attack-but now it can be done within 6 hours. So doctors can give fast care to those who need it and send the others home.

What Are the Tests for Coronary Heart Disease?

Diagnostic tests are usually needed to confirm the presence and assess the severity of coronary heart disease. Your doctor will know whether you need any of them. Often more than one test is needed because different tests supply different information. Also, patients vary in their symptoms and so may need more than one test to find out the heart's condition.

The main tests used to diagnose coronary heart disease are described below. Many are not "invasive" procedures—they are done outside the body—and are painless.

The tests are:

Electrocardiogram (ECG or EKG) makes a graphic record of the heart's electrical activity as it beats. This can show abnormal heartbeats, muscle damage, blood flow problems, and heart enlargement.

Stress test (or treadmill test or exercise ECG) records the ECG during exercise, usually on a treadmill or exercise bicycle. Some heart problems show up only when more effort is asked of the heart, as happens during increased activity. So the exercise ECG may be done even if the resting ECG is normal.

Other exercise tests may be done with an ECG or a nuclear scan to assess heart muscle contraction or blood flow in the heart.

Older women may not be able to exercise due to arthritis or another condition. For them, a stress test can be done without exercise by using a drug that increases blood flow.

143

Echocardiography converts sound waves, bounced off the heart, into images that show heart size, shape, and movement. The sound waves also can be used to see how much blood is pumped out by the heart when it contracts.

Nuclear scan assesses heart muscle contraction as blood flows through the heart. A small amount of radioactive material is injected into a vein, usually in the arm, and a scanning camera then records how much is taken up by the heart muscle.

Coronary angiography (or arteriography) displays blood flow problems and blockages. A fine, flexible tube (or "catheter") is threaded through an artery of an arm or leg up into the heart. A fluid that shows up on x-ray is then injected, and the heart and blood vessels are filmed as the heart pumps. The picture is called an angiogram or arteriogram.

Treating Your Heart Right

You can reduce your risk of complications of coronary heart disease. But you must do your part.

There are three main types of treatment: lifestyle, medication, and special procedures for advanced atherosclerosis. A discussion of each of these follows.

Lifestyle

Since you have coronary heart disease, you will need to take five key steps to keep your heart as healthy as possible: stop smoking, lower high blood pressure, lower high blood cholesterol, lose any extra weight, and become physically active.

In fact, these steps are so crucial for good health that they should be adopted by all people, even the young. So as a plus, do them with your family and friends. Studies show that such support makes lifestyle changes easier. You'll improve more if others join you in your new behavior. And teaching your children or grandchildren heart-healthy habits is a gift that will last them a lifetime.

Stop Smoking Cigarettes

There is no safe way to smoke. Smoking accelerates atherosclerosis. If you smoke, you are two to six times more likely to have a heart attack than a nonsmoker, and your risk increases with the number of cigarettes you smoke each day.

But if you quit, then the risk to your heart drops sharply, even in the first year, no matter what your age.

Even if you've had a heart attack, you'll benefit from quitting—some women's risk of having a second heart attack is cut by 50 percent or more after they stop smoking.

The National Heart, Lung, and Blood Institute (NHLBI) has information to help you kick the habit or ask your doctor for advice.

Lower High Blood Pressure

Also called hypertension, high blood pressure usually has no symptoms. It has no cure but can and must be controlled. High blood pressure makes the heart work harder and, uncontrolled, can lead to heart disease, stroke, heart failure, kidney problems, and other conditions.

Blood pressure is given as two numbers—the systolic pressure over the diastolic pressure, and both are important. A measurement of 140/90 mmHg or above means you have high blood pressure. But even pressures slightly under that can put our heart at greater risk.

Most American women over age 60 have high blood pressure—nearly 80 percent of black women over age 60 have it.

However, blood pressure does not have to increase with age—hypertension can be prevented. And controlling our blood pressure will reduce your chance of suffering a first or repeat heart attack. Discuss your blood pressure with your doctor.

A normal blood pressure level is around 120/80. Often, this can be reached through lifestyle changes. If necessary, a medication will be used. If a drug is prescribed, you must take it as instructed, even if you feel fine because, if you' stop, your blood pressure probably will rise again. If you make lifestyle changes, however, your doctor may be able to decrease your medication.

The lifestyle steps that prevent and control high blood pressure are: losing excess weight, becoming physically active, choosing foods low in salt and sodium, and limiting alcohol intake.

Salt and sodium both affect blood pressure and must be watched. Salt (sodium chloride) is only one source of sodium, and there are others. You should consume no more than 6 grams (about 1 teaspoon) of salt a day, which equals 2.4 grains of sodium. This includes ALL salt—that in processed foods or added in cooking or at the table. A good way to keep track of sodium is by reading food labels.

If you drink alcohol, you should have no more than one drink a day. One drink equals 1.5 ounces of 80-proof whiskey, or 5 ounces of wine, or 12 ounces of beer (regular or light).

Recently, news stories have said that alcohol may lower the risk of having a heart attack. But this has yet to be proved. And too much alcohol has dangers. So if you don't drink, it's best not to start.

Lower High Blood Cholesterol

Why is cholesterol so important? The body makes all the cholesterol it needs. Extra cholesterol and fat in the diet cause the atherosclerotic buildup inside blood vessels. So, high blood cholesterol leads to coronary heart disease.

And, once you have coronary heart disease, an elevated blood cholesterol increases your risk of a future heart attack. But you can take steps to keep your blood cholesterol from rising.

Cholesterol travels through the blood in protein-fat packages called lipoproteins. The two main types are: low-density lipoprotein, or LDL, which causes deposits and is termed the "bad" cholesterol; and high-density lipoprotein, or HDL, which helps remove cholesterol from the blood and is referred to as the "good" cholesterol.

Women who have coronary heart disease should have an LDL level of 100 mg/dL or less. A low level of HDL (less than 35 mg/dL) is a major risk factor for coronary heart disease. Physical activity, weight loss if you're overweight, and stopping smoking help raise the level of HDL.

Women with coronary heart disease need to have a "lipoprotein analysis" done to check their levels of total cholesterol, HDL, and LDL, as well as triglycerides, which is another type of fat in the bloodstream. Lipoprotein tests should be taken on two occasions and the results averaged. The level of LDL is usually the main target of treatment.

Many women with coronary heart disease can lower their high blood cholesterol enough through lifestyle changes. However, cholesterol-lowering drugs may be needed as well. Hormone replacement therapy also may improve blood cholesterol.

The lifestyle changes call for adopting a healthy eating plan, becoming physically active, and losing excess weight (the latter two described below). For healthy eating, have:

- Less than 7 percent of your day's total calories from saturated fat

- 30 percent or less of your day's total calories from fat

- Less than 200 milligrams of dietary cholesterol a day

- Just enough calories a day to achieve and maintain a healthy weight

Foods high in total fat and in saturated fat are also high in calories and often in cholesterol. Saturated fat, which raises blood cholesterol more than anything else in the diet, is found mainly in foods that come from animals—dairy products, meat, and poultry skin. Some vegetable fats—coconut oil, cocoa butter, palm kernel oil, and palm oil-also are high in saturated fat. Cholesterol is found only in foods that come from animals—egg yolks, liver, and kidney, for example.

A few pointers: To cut down on saturated fat, total fat, and cholesterol, choose fish, poultry, and lean cuts of meat; choose low-fat foods; choose low-fat or no-fat milk and other dairy products; and eat plenty of fruits and vegetables. Breads, rice, and pasta made from enriched or whole grains also are good choices. Broil, bake, roast, or poach, instead of frying, and be sure any sauce is also low in fat.

Lose Excess Weight

America is becoming heftier—and older women are among those gaining weight. More than half of American women ages 50 to 59 are overweight—30 years ago, only 35 percent of them were. This is a dangerous trend, because being overweight increases the risk of coronary heart disease, even if there are no other risk factors.

But being overweight also increases the chance of developing several other risk factors, which would compound the danger.

Losing excess weight is critical for good health. But weight loss must be viewed as a change of lifestyle, not as a temporary effort to drop pounds quickly. Such quick fixes are just that—temporary. The weight soon returns.

To lose weight, follow a heart-healthy eating plan and become physically active. Eat a variety of low-calorie, nutritious foods in moderate amounts. Keep to the eating pattern outlined for high blood cholesterol. Do not try to lose more than one-half to one pound a week.

Remember: When it comes to weight loss, take it slow and steady—learn a new way of eating to get to and stay at a healthy weight.

Become Physically Active

Physical activity is one of the best ways to control coronary heart disease. It is vital for good health and well being. It helps lower LDL and raise HDL. Even if you're overweight, you'll have a lower blood pressure if you're active. You may worry that "becoming physically active" requires a lot of time and effort. Not so. Research shows that even a little exercise can improve your heart's health. And "exercise" can mean going up a flight of stairs (instead of taking the elevator) or gardening or walking at the mall. Walk with a friend or your husband, or get your whole family moving together.

Try to do some type of activity for at least 30 minutes on most days. But, if 30 minutes is too long a period, break up the time into shorter sessions done throughout the day. Incorporate exercise into your other daily activities too.

Since you have coronary heart disease, you should consult with your doctor before starting a physical activity program. This is especially important if you're over age 55, have been inactive, or have diabetes or another medical problem. Your doctor can help you prevent problems from overexertion.

It also is important to exercise in a way that will help you without hurting you. If you've been inactive, start slowly. Walking 10-15 minutes, three times a week, makes a good start.

If you've had a heart attack, you'll benefit greatly from exercise. Many hospitals have a "cardiac" (heart) rehabilitation program. Ask your doctor about your ability to exercise and about a suitable program for you.

If you have arthritis or another limiting condition, you may benefit from exercises that help keep you as flexible and healthy as possible. Again, ask your doctor about a suitable exercise.

Medications

A healthy lifestyle will improve your heart's condition. But you may need medication too, especially if you have chest pain, or if you have high blood pressure or high blood cholesterol that was not lowered enough with lifestyle changes.

Drugs can have side effects, so none should be taken without first seeing your doctor. If you take a drug, follow the dose instructions carefully and report any troublesome side effects to your doctor. Often a change in dose or type of drug can stop the side effect. Your doctor may even prescribe a combination of drugs to treat your coronary heart disease.

The following list will briefly introduce you to some medications used to treat coronary heart disease and its risk factors. If you need a medication, discuss it with your doctor and be sure you understand bow and why it should be taken.

- **Aspirin**—helps prevent heart attacks when taken regularly in a low dose on a doctor's orders.

- **Digitalis**—makes the heart contract harder and is used when the heart's pumping function has been weakened; it also slows some fast heart rhythms.

- **ACE inhibitor**—stops production of a chemical that makes blood vessels narrow and is used for high blood pressure and heart muscle that has been damaged.

- **Beta-blocker**—reduces how hard the heart must work and is used for high blood pressure, chest pain, and to prevent a repeat heart attack.

- **Nitrate (including nitroglycerine)**—relaxes blood vessels and alleviates chest pain.

- **Calcium-channel blocker**—relaxes blood vessels; used for high blood pressure and chest pain.

- **Diuretic**—decreases fluid in the body and is used for high blood pressure.

- **Blood cholesterol-lowering agents**—HMG CoA reductase inhibitors (or "statins"), nicotinic acid, bile acid sequestrants, fibric acid derivatives, and probucol.

Special Procedures

If you have advanced atherosclerosis, you may need a special procedure to open an artery and improve blood flow. This is usually done to ease severe chest pain or clear major or multiple blockages in blood vessels.

The two main procedures are:

- **Coronary angioplasty**—also called "balloon" angioplasty. A fine tube is threaded through an artery to the narrowed heart vessel, where a tiny balloon at its tip is inflated. The balloon flattens the buildup and stretches the artery, improving blood flow. It is then deflated and removed, along with the tube.

- **Coronary artery bypass graft surgery**—also known as "bypass surgery." A piece of blood vessel is taken from the leg or chest and is stitched onto the narrowed heart artery, making a bypass around the blockage. Sometimes, more than one bypass is needed.

Bypass surgery is used when blockages in an artery can't be reached by, or are too long or hard for, angioplasty. A bypass requires about 1 week in the hospital and several weeks of recuperation at home.

Factors that Put Your Heart at Risk

One in ten American women ages 45 to 64 has some form of heart disease. That increases to one in five for women over age 65. Some of the factors that increase the risk to your heart cannot be controlled—but most can. You'll protect your heart by controlling those that can be changed.

Here's a rundown of both types of risk factors:

Unchangeable Risk Factors

• Being age 55 or older

• Having a family history of early heart disease (this means having a mother or sister who has been diagnosed with heart disease before age 65, or a father or brother diagnosed before age 55).

Changeable Risk Factors

• Cigarette smoking

• High blood pressure

• High blood cholesterol

• Overweight

• Physical inactivity

• Diabetes

Talking with Your Doctor

Caring for a chronic condition like coronary heart disease is a partnership—you and your doctor should work as a team. That means good communication. Here are some pointers to help you talk with your doctor:

Before Your Office Visit

• Write down your concerns.

- Keep a diary of your symptoms, so you can describe them accurately.

- Note any past treatments.

- Gather any drugs you are taking and bring them or a list of them to the office visit.

During Your Office Visit

- **Be open.** You will only hurt yourself if you're not. For instance, if you have trouble breathing or have pain, tell your doctor.

- **Briefly describe all symptoms.** Tell when each started, how often it happens, and if it has been getting worse.

- **Note any causes of stress in your life.** For instance, say if you are the caregiver for a sick parent or husband, or have other stressful responsibilities.

- **Ask questions.** Be sure you understand what the doctor says. Ask for an explanation of any term you do not understand. Be sure you know the instructions for any medication—when to take it; what to do if you forget and skip a dose; what other drug, food, or activity to avoid while taking it; and what side effects may occur with it.

- **Write notes.** This will help you remember what the doctor says.

- **Bring a friend or relative with you if necessary.** If you are worried about understanding what the doctor says or have trouble hearing, have someone with you during the discussion.

- **Share your views.** If something bothers you, say so. The doctor needs to know if something is working or not, or if you're having trouble following a treatment. For instance, if you're having trouble fixing low-saturated fat meals, say so. You may be referred to a dietitian for help. Dietitians are health care professionals who can help design an eating plan for you.

If a Diagnostic Test Is Ordered

- Ask the reason and find out what will be learned from the test.
- Ask when results will be ready.
- Know what the test involves and how to get ready for it.
- Ask who will do the test.

- Find out if you will need help getting home after the test.

- Find out if the test poses any dangers or side effects.

If You Need a Special Procedure

- Find out the benefits and risks of the procedure.

- Ask what kind of doctor you need for it and get a referral.

- Ask if you will need to be hospitalized and for how long.

- Ask what kind of pain or discomfort you may feel.

- Ask about the recovery period, how long it will last, and what it will involve.

Diabetes—The Self-Help Disease

Diabetes mellitus increases the risk to your heart. It also is the single most common cause of kidney disease.

If you have diabetes, you will need to control it. Because those with it must manage their condition day-by-day, diabetes is sometimes called the "self-help disease."

In diabetes, the body cannot properly convert foods into energy. This causes a buildup in the blood of a form of sugar called glucose. The buildup produces symptoms and damages organs.

Women should have a routine test for diabetes. The doctor will test for too much sugar in the urine or blood.

Symptoms of diabetes include: a vague sick feeling, being "run down," increased thirst, frequent urination, unexplained weight loss, blurred vision, skin infections or itching, and slow healing of cuts, bruises, and gum and urinary tract infections.

Controlling diabetes can help keep your heart healthy. For more information on diabetes, contact:

National Diabetes Information Clearinghouse
Box NDIC
9000 Rockville Pike
Bethesda, MD 20892
(301) 654-3327

Tips for Having Your Blood Pressure Taken

A blood pressure test is painless. Here are some tips to assure that you get a good reading:

- Before the test, sit for 5 minutes with your feet flat on the ground, arm resting on a table at the level of your heart
- Wear short sleeves so your arm is exposed
- If you know your arm requires a large adult cuff, say so
- Get two readings, taken at least 2 minutes apart, and average the results

For More Information

The NHLBI has more information that can help you improve your heart health. Materials cover such topics as: how to stop smoking, high blood cholesterol, high blood pressure, physical activity, heart-healthy recipes, hormone replacement therapy, coronary heart disease, heart failure, and heart arrhythmias.

Contact:

NHLBI Information Center
P.O. Box 30105
Bethesda, MD 20824-0105
Phone: (301) 251-1222
Tollfree: (800) 575-WELL.

Chapter 22

Women and Heart Attacks

Despite the common view that it is a male health problem, heart disease kills more women than men in America[1]. As a woman ages, the risk of heart attack increases as does the likelihood of death and disability from heart attack. The advances in prevention, diagnosis, treatment, and rehabilitation associated with better outcomes have been developed on research whose sampling bias has favored male subjects. Although the disease is an equal opportunity killer, women may not equally have access to or benefit from the prevention, early diagnosis, treatment, and rehabilitation strategies that have helped so many men[2].

Primary care practitioners can reduce the needless death and disability that result from this traditional gender bias. Health promotion interventions geared toward risk identification, awareness, and reduction are at least as important as the routine screening tests[3-4]. Astute practitioners can recognize subtle changes in the presentation of angina, or atypical symptoms that signal a myocardial infarction (MI) or unstable angina in women. Further, primary care practitioners are in a position to help women gain access to the same appropriate testing, referrals, treatment, and follow-up care that men receive.

"Women and heart attacks: prevention, diagnosis, and care," used with permission from P. M. Arnstein, E. F. Buselli, and S.H. Rankin, *The Nurse Practitioner*, May 1996, Vol. 21, No. 5, Pg. 57-69, © Springhouse Corporation.

Magnitude of the Problem

Cardiovascular disease is the leading cause of death in America, regardless of gender. For women, it accounts for 2.5 million hospitalizations and half a million deaths a year[2]. There is growing evidence that once in the hospital, women receive substandard care more often than men[5-7]. Women can suffer an MI at any stage of adult life, although on average they are 10 years older than their male counterparts. Women narrow the gap after menopause, and by age 75 the incidence of coronary heart disease in women exceeds that of men[1,6].

Part of the reason women are believed to have fewer heart attacks is that they are often not diagnosed when an MI has occurred. Of those in the Framingham Study who have had heart attacks, 38% of women (compared with 27% of men) had an MI that went unrecognized[3]. The predictive value of the standard diagnostic tests are lower in women[2] and once diagnosed, they are often treated less aggressively[8]. Death rates for women after MI are higher than for men, whether the death occurs in the hospital[7,9], within 6 months[10-11], at 1 year[12], or in the years that follow[13-14]. These studies indicate that women have a three-times higher death rate than men both in the hospital and at 1 year after an MI. Those women who do survive are more likely to be disabled or unable to participate in cardiac rehabilitation programs[2].

Primary Prevention

Nonmodifiable Risks

Advancing age, race, and family history are considered nonmodifiable risk factors. The current cardiopulmonary resuscitation (CPR) courses that are widely taught to lay and professional groups still list the male gender as a nonmodifiable risk factor[15]; this may foster an unwarranted sense of security in women.

Age is considered a powerful independent risk factor for the increased incidence, morbidity, and mortality associated with MI, regardless of gender[5,10,12-13, 16-17]. In fact, many investigators have discounted the presence of a gender bias because, when the influence of age is removed, the differences between men and women are reportedly insignificant[10,12,17-18]. Other investigators confirm that despite differences in age, the female gender is a significant predictor of death and disability from heart attacks[5,9,13,16].

Race has been associated with relative risk of heart disease prevalence and mortality. African-Americans have a higher prevalence of heart disease than whites. African-American women have the highest rate of nonfatal types of coronary disease, with twice the rate of angina as white women and five times that of white men[19]. African-American women have close to a 50% mortality rate from MI, nearly double that of African-American men, compared with 32% for white women and 23% mortally for white men[20]. Among Asian-Americans, South Asians have a higher relative risk (3.7 times), and Chinese have a lower (0.6 times) relative risk of ischemic heart disease when compared with whites. However, after emigrating to America, Japanese, Filipinos, and other Asian-Americans had comparable risks of ischemic heart disease as whites[21]. This raises questions whether this risk is related to race, ethnicity, culture, or diet.

Family history of an MI by a first-degree relative is considered an important risk factor[15]. A large-scale longitudinal study indicated that this risk is significant only as a predictor of premature (before age 55) coronary heart disease, and is a stronger predictor among women than men[22]. First-degree relatives of women who died from coronary heart disease before age 55 were more than five times as likely to have early coronary disease than control family members. Their daughters incurred nearly twice the risk of coronary heart disease than their sons[23]. Despite knowledge of familial risks, their progeny have failed to engage in risk-reduction behavior[24].

Modifiable Risk Factors

Primary care practitioners can positively influence health in the area of modifiable risk factors, including lifestyle changes, cholesterol reduction, co-morbidity management, and attention to psychosocial factors.

Lifestyle. Lifestyle modification of risks (e.g., diet, exercise, and smoking) is considered to be as important as the dramatic treatment advances during the 1970s in explaining the decline of morbidity and mortality from MIs in the past 2 decades[25]. Cigarette smoking (including passive smoking), however, is the greatest single cause of preventable death in America[15]. Women who have heart attacks before age 40 are almost always smokers and older women who smoke are at five-times greater risk for sudden death than women who don't smoke[6]. Women who stop smoking can realize a 50% to 80% reduction in their risk of coronary disease within 5 years of quitting[26].

Smoking-related risks are compounded for young women when other risk factors (e.g., obesity or sedentary lifestyle) are present or when estrogen is being used for contraception[27-29]. The effects of smoking, which increases platelet aggregability, fibrinogen activity[30], cholesterol levels, and triglyceride levels[31], increase the woman's risk of both heart attack and stroke. Despite the known risks associated with cigarette smoke, more young women smoke today than young men, possibly because smoking is used to control weight[6].

Women with more upper body fat (as measured by waist to hip ratio) are at greater risk for heart disease. Wing and associates question whether this is a direct effect or related to other known risk factors[28]. High correlations were found between women with more upper body fat and such factors as higher blood pressure, cholesterol, anxiety, anger, depression, and smoking.

Upper body fat is also associated with lower levels of high-density lipoprotein and less perceived social support. These factors remain significant even after controlling for body mass[28]. The primary care practitioner should discuss the known risks with all women, regardless of their "apple, pear, or carrot shape," to identify opportunities for improvement, set goals, and reinforce healthy lifestyle patterns. Weight loss, a low-fat diet, smoking cessation, stress management, and regular exercise make up the healthy lifestyle that is believed to reduce cardiac risk, primarily by significantly reducing serum cholesterol[32].

Cholesterol. Lipid abnormalities influence coronary artery disease development in both men and women. Holme analyzed 19 research reports, each with 100 to 50,000 people studied. His analysis found that each 1% reduction in cholesterol corresponded to a 2% reduction in the risk of cardiac disease[32]. More than two-thirds of those studies excluded women despite known gender differences, and thus the extent of benefit women realize by reducing their cholesterol remains unclear. Of the observational studies done on women, 90% indicate that as total cholesterol rises, so does the risk of coronary heart disease[26], supporting the importance of managing cholesterol levels in women.

Early in life women have higher high-density lipoprotein (HDL) levels and lower low-density lipoprotein (LDL) levels than men, both of which are strongly associated with a lower risk of heart attacks[26,33]. At menopause, however, women's LDLs and triglyceride levels generally increase, so that by age 55 they exceed those of men. These increases are strong independent risk factors for heart attacks in women[26,34].

158

Menopause is believed to affect lipids by decreasing circulation of women's own estrogens. Before menopause however, estrogen-containing oral contraceptives raise cholesterol, LDLs, and triglycerides while lowering HDLs[33,35]. These undesired effects are similar to changes in lipids noted by premenopausal smokers[31]. The relative risk of having a heart attack as the result of taking oral contraceptives is believed insignificant, unless the women also smoke[26]. After menopause, oral estrogen has the desired effect of raising HDLs and lowering LDLs[33]. Hormone replacement therapy using estrogen, with or without added progestin, has been shown to significantly reduce the risk of coronary disease in large-scale studies representing geographically and culturally diverse groups of postmenopausal women[27,36-39]. A review of over 30 observational studies suggests that replacement estrogen increases HDLs and reduces LDLs by as much as 15%, resulting in a 44% reduction in the risk of coronary heart disease in women after menopause[26].

Studies done predominantly on men suggest that serum cholesterol levels can be reduced by as much as 20% by diet, weight loss, and exercise[40]. These methods are less effective in lowering cholesterol for women than men[41]; thus estrogen replacement therapy may be used in combination with these lifestyle changes to reduce or delay the need for lipid-lowering drugs.

Co-morbidities. Co-morbidities that increase the risk of MI in women include hypertension, hyperlipidemia, diabetes, congestive heart failure, and obesity[6,14,16]. Although the risks of developing coronary artery disease with hyperthyroidism have not been calculated, generalized cardiac effects of this primarily female disease are known. Co-morbidities such as arthritis, peptic ulcer, or chronic lung disease do not have known relationships to heart disease; however, their symptoms may contribute to delays or a missed diagnosis when a heart attack has occurred.

Hypertension and hyperlipidemia are the most consistent risk factors for predicting cardiovascular diseases in women over 35 years old[14]. Of the women who had heart attacks, 29% were found to have preexisting angina, diabetes, or hypertension. Those with diabetes are at particularly high risk for dying if they do have a heart attack[25]. This association with preexisting heart disease or other co-morbidities is significantly stronger in women than men[6,17-18,42-43]. It is assumed that effective management (secondary prevention) of these disorders will reduce the related risk.

Psychosocial factors. Psychosocial factors are believed to contribute to heart disease. The extent that stress contributes to heart disease in women is not currently clear. The psychosocial profile for women is not the high-status, high-stress picture normally associated with cardiovascular risk in men. Women employed in pink-collar occupations, with low control and little power (e.g., secretaries and clerks), are twice as likely to develop coronary artery disease than women working in white-collar jobs[44]. Women who have careers and maintain the role of wife and mother have better cardiac health than those who occupy fewer roles[45]. Another interesting contrast is that stress is significantly elevated in women who work more than 10 hours a week in overtime and reduced in men[46].

Factors Affecting Morbidity and Mortality

Women have more complications and higher mortality rates than their male counterparts from the time they are diagnosed with coronary heart disease until several years after their MI. The reasons for this are not clear. However, the current delays in seeking care, misdiagnosis, and the less-aggressive treatment of women probably contribute to these higher rates. These need to be corrected before other strategies can be investigated.

Morbidity

Angina is the first symptom of heart disease in 56% of women compared with 43% of men. African-American women have an even higher prevalence of angina than Anglo-American women[47]. Women are more likely to experience nonobstructive variant angina (at rest with reversible ST-segment elevation) than men[48-49]. This nonobstructive form of angina has the advantage of lower associated mortality rates but the disadvantage of more false-negative diagnostic tests and less responsiveness to pain relief treatments[48]. The rate of women with unstable angina or silent ischemia also exceeds that of men. Still, some professionals fail to believe women's reports of pain even though 75% of women with angina have evidence of significant myocardial ischemia when tested[48].

Women also have non-Q wave (subendocardial) MIs more often than men, which puts them at risk for a higher rate of re-infarction[20,50]. This may explain why 29% of women have a second heart attack during hospitalization, compared with a 12% re-infarction rate in men. This trend continues during the first postinfarction year when 40%

of women, compared with 13% of men have re-infarctions[20]. These nonobstructive, non-Q wave MIs may contribute to the undertreatment or underrepresentation of women in research protocols as they fail to meet the eligibility criteria.

Mortality

Fewer women (34% versus 50% in men) present with MI as the first symptom of heart disease. However, 68% of women (compared with 49% of men) have a fatal MI without prior symptoms of heart disease. More women ages 35-44 and substantially more women over 75 years die from heart disease than men of the same age[48].

The most significant predictors of death in both men and women are the extent of heart damage as measured by the degree of heart failure by Killip class (1=no failure to 4=cardiogenic shock), ejection fractions (less than 35%), and the presence of co-morbidities[10]. Additional factors associated with higher mortality rates that are more prevalent in women include such complications as stroke, heart failure, cardiac rupture, depression, and less social support[10,51-52]. In fact, patients with two or more sources of emotional support (e.g., spouse or confidant) were three times more likely to survive 5 years than those who had no one. Women who are alone, are confined to home, have persistent unrelieved symptoms, and have difficulty with household tasks are most vulnerable[53]. Provisions for outside support made by the practitioner may enhance survival.

Practitioners can perhaps have the greatest impact on mortality by reducing the time from the onset of symptoms to effective treatment by convincing women that they are at risk and that it is important to seek help expediently.

In Rankin's study of African-American and Anglo-American women, there was an average delay of 10 hours from the presentation of symptoms to arrival at the emergency department[54]. Thus many were not eligible for thrombolysis. The absence of classical chest pain in these women contributed to missed diagnosis, which then contributed to the tragic disability and needless death of women with heart attacks[54-55].

Pathophysiology

The process of coronary artery damage, thrombosis, and platelet aggregation often progresses until there is a total occlusion of one or more coronary arteries. The expanding area of ischemia, injury, and

161

necrosis results in irreversible myocardial damage within 6 hours. This process is believed to be the same regardless of gender[50,56]; however, women do have more nonocclusive forms of the disease.

Since women are often elderly when they experience an MI, age-related physiology may be relevant. Increased density, sclerosis, or calcification of the blood vessels, myocardium, and heart valves reduces the responsiveness and efficiency of the cardiovascular system. Heart murmurs, abnormal heart rates, irregular rhythms, and reduction in cardiac output often occur[57-58]. Angina in the elderly is less typically in the substernal location, often nonexertional, less severe in intensity, and not as responsive to nitroglycerin when compared with the younger population[59]. Nonangina symptoms, such as indigestion, dyspnea, exacerbation of congestive heart failure, and confusion, may signal an MI in the elderly population[59].

Anatomically, women generally have smaller rib cages, heart muscles, and coronary lumens than men[60]. Osteoporosis and kyphosis change the shape of the thorax and may produce an anatomic emphysema[58]. Women's breast tissue may further add complexity to diagnosis by serving as the site for referred pain, or interfere with assessment and diagnostic procedures. These changes make evaluating the subtle (but significant) physical changes challenging to even the best diagnostician.

The pain associated with angina pectoris is believed due to the production of lactic acid by ischemic muscle, which chemically stimulates pain fibers[56]. This description may be challenged because the heart is innervated by the glossopharyngeal and the vagus nerve (9th and 10th cranial nerves), which are neither designed to carry messages of pain, nor connect directly with pain pathways in the spine or brain[61]. This form of "visceral pain" is by nature vague, sickening and difficult to describe or locate[62]. Since visceral pain is not yet understood completely in the animal model, it will likely be several years before the differences between male and female patterns of angina can be satisfactorily explained.

Symptoms

Although physical, emotional, and environmental stress are often considered factors that can precipitate an MI, 83% of women develop infarctions while at rest[6]. The typical presentation of angina in men is described as a pressure, heaviness, or tightness in the chest that radiates to the neck, jaw, or arm. It is usually relieved by rest and sublingual nitroglycerin. Only 24% of women with MI in a recent study presented with this classic description of chest pain[54]. Table 22.1 lists the atypical presenting symptoms as described by women in interviews after their MI. Other symptoms, such as nausea, diaphoresis, weakness, fatigue, and blood pressure aberrations, may signal an MI with or without angina[16]. This suggests that primary care practitioners should consider the diagnosis of MI in women even when chest pain is not present. It also demands that practitioners listen carefully to what women say as well as clarify what is implied but not said. Table 22.2 delineates functional health patterns that are relevant to a woman's cardiovascular health and should be considered while obtaining a history.

Making the Diagnosis

The presence of any suspicious signs and symptoms (see Tables 22.1 and 22.3) compels the practitioner to rule out MI. In addition to documenting baseline and repeat measures of vital signs (including a pain assessment), a 12-lead electrocardiogram (ECG) should be done

Table 22.1. Atypical Presenting Symptoms Reported by Women and the Onset of a Heart Attack(*)

- Epigastric pain
- Chest cramping
- "Flutters" without pain
- Shortness of breath
- Lower abdominal pain
- Severe fatigue
- Tiredness, depression
- Epigastric burning
- Dull pain between breasts
- Bilateral arm pain half an hour before chest pain
- Sudden shortness of breath, unable to talk move or breathe
- Bilateral posterior shoulder pain
- Ankle edema, rapid weight gain
- Thoughts of death

(*) Examples of MI presenting symptoms were reported in interviews of Anglo-American and African-American women participating in Dr. S. Rankin's study (R55 NR02617).

Table 22.2. History by functional health patterns, health perception/ health management, chief concern, past history and history of current problem, medications and pattern of use, perceived cardiac risk factors, COLDERR assessment (Character, Onset, Location, Duration, Exacerbation, Relief, Radiation) of discomforts, and intensity (0=none, 10=worst) of discomfort.

Nutrition/Metabolic

Type of diet.

Association of discomfort to eating.

Volume and frequency of alcohol or caffeinated beverage consumption.

Nutritional problems (including being overweight or undernourished) and knowledge of desirable nutrition.

Thyroid or other metabolic disorders.

Elimination

Frequency of urination.

Ankle edema or dyspnea.

Symptoms during bowel movements.

Activity/Exercise

Types, frequency, duration, and tolerance of activities.

Symptoms before, during, or after activities.

Regularity of exercise or activities.

Physical setup of home (e.g., stairs).

Sleep/Rest

Usual sleep pattern.

Presence of daytime fatigue, nocturnal dyspnea, or orthopnea.

Preferred method of relaxation.

Cognitive/Perceptual

Patient's perception of what the problem is and what is needed.

Knowledge of presenting symptoms and importance of seeking help expediently.

Information desired about cardiac health.

Table 22.2. (continued)

Roles/Relationships

Living situation and important people in their current life (e.g., spouse, children, neighbors, friends).

Satisfaction with support received.

Need for additional support or counseling.

Sexual/Reproductive

Current level of sexual activity.

Symptoms during sex.

Hormones replacement therapy.

Stress/Coping

Rate intensity of current stress (0=none, 10=worst).

Symptoms associated with stress.

Stress-reduction techniques.

Sources of stress.

Self-Perception/Self-Concept

Recent changes in mood or personality.

Perceived reason for change.

Values/Beliefs

Objects of meaning and value in life.

Beliefs about what is needed to be in a satisfactory health state.

Motivators to change health behavior.

Suspicious Signs

Short of obvious signs of distress (e.g., pain behaviors, dyspnea, or unresponsiveness), there are some subtle signs that may be indicative of cardiac ischemia that the astute practitioner can perceive.

Confusion, fatigue, anxiety, or agitation are easily discounted as associated with emotional state, personality trait, or simply related to old age.

Table 22.3. Suspicious Signs of MI with Special Consideration for Women

Assessment	*Signs*	*Considerations for Women*
Inspection.	Pallor, jugular venous distension, dyspnea and edema. Point of maximal impulse (PMI) may reveal a dyskinetic precordial heave.	Breast tissue may precule visualization of the PMI.
Percussion.	Percussion of the cardiac borders may reveal an enlarged heart or mass, but contributes little to the evaluation of coronary artery patency.	Breast tissue interference. Women have smaller hearts than men when healthy and less hypertrophy when ill.
Palpation.	Right ventricular precordial impulse in late diastole is the only palpable sign of cardiac disease. Palpation of peripheral pulses indirectly assesses hardening of arteries, but doesn't accurately advise the practitioner of lumen patency.	Breast tissue may render trills or pulses less palpable.
Auscultation.	A fourth heart sound S_4 is audible in almost all patients with acute ischemia. The third heart sound S_3, like the fourth, is best heard at apex during inspiration. S_3 is usually associated with a massive MI. New heart murmer signals heart disease. Pericardial friction rub at the sternal border. Bibasilar crackles with abnormal heart sounds favors the diagnosis of coronary heart disease.	May result from normal aging heart. Breast tissue may interfere with auscultation. Thoracic change associated with aging may also interfere. Women are less likely to develop a pericardial friction rub than men post-MI.

as soon as possible. If the condition warrants, emergency treatment and continuous monitoring are initiated per local protocol.

During the diagnostic work-up, the practitioner should recall that any symptom or noninvasive test has less predictive value in women than men[48]. Further, women tend to have: non-Q wave infarctions[9]; more atrial fibrillation, supraventricular tachycardia and heart blocks; less ventricular ectopy[64]; and false-positive ECG exercise tests (very few false-negatives). Many of the newer radionuclide studies need to be further analyzed to clarify their usefulness in women; however the exercise radionuclide ventriculography test has poor diagnostic value in women and should be avoided[48].

Implications for Practice

Implications for practice include primary prevention-oriented interventions, diagnostic considerations, and rehabilitation guidelines. Each is discussed in the following section with particular attention given to differences between men and women.

Primary Prevention

Utilization of primary prevention principles involves health teaching for all age-groups. Since women are the chief health educators in households, young women need instruction regarding the importance of low-fat, low-calorie diets after their children are 2 years old. At the same time, they need to be advised of their own future risk of coronary artery disease (CAD) in much the same way that young women are taught to consider risk factors for breast cancer. The importance of exercise as a means of decreasing obesity and stress is also within the purview of the practitioner's teaching regarding CAD.

Rankin's recent article may explain why the current group of older women experiencing MI are least likely to have engaged in health promotion activities earlier in life[54]. For example, information regarding cigarette smoking and appropriate dietary information was not available to women when they were young and establishing health-related lifestyles. Thus today's women with CAD and MI may have amended their eating patterns but prior behavior may have already established atherosclerosis. Likewise, the women who are now suffering CAD and MI were less likely to engage in vigorous exercise when they were younger when compared with the young women of today.

Therefore, older women may not profit from primary prevention interventions to the same extent as younger women. Younger women, and their offspring, will benefit, however, if primary health care providers can educate them about the importance of smoking cessation, limiting fat intake, and regular aerobic exercise.

Diagnostic Considerations

Once women have been apprised of their risk of CAD and MI they need to be taught the symptoms that signify the need for medical attention. In addition to the symptoms commonly experienced by men, women may have accompanying shortness of breath, nonclassic chest pain, or epigastric distress[54]. The importance of considering other than midsternal discomfort as symptomatic of CAD and MI is underlined by the long delay before women present for treatment. Women should be taught that the faster they report their symptoms to their provider, the greater the possibility of limiting cardiac damage.

Because health care providers have disregarded women's symptoms in the past, it is crucial that the practitioner teach women to advocate for themselves in medical situations, and, if necessary, assist in the advocacy process. Women need to know that many health care providers will take their complaints seriously and not write them off as hypochondriacs as has been noted in past research[65].

If women are at risk for MI because of modifiable and non-modifiable risk factors, family members, significant others and paraprofessional health care providers, such as emergency medical technicians, should also be included in teaching related to symptomatology. Women experiencing acute MI accompanied by epigastric pain, nausea and vomiting, and shortness of breath are not in a good position to advocate for themselves.

Rehabilitation

The practitioner must be aggressive in suggesting rehabilitation activities. Only a very small percentage of women experiencing MI are likely to engage in structured cardiac rehabilitative exercise for health restoration, a fact that most likely results from cohort influences in the group of women currently experiencing MI. These women were not socialized to competitive activities, exercising in the company of men, or to "working up a sweat," thus they are frequently uncomfortable in standard cardiac rehabilitation services.

Rankin's work demonstrates that women are slower to return to physical activity than men[54]. For example, at 6 weeks post-MI only 57% were walking two level blocks outdoors. The slower return to activity levels may be related to their preexisting co-morbidities, which limit activity levels. On the other hand, women may not receive specific information that is tailored to their own exercise tolerance levels or to realistic exercise performance and preferences. Women often have less transportation, encouragement, and support from their spouses than men after MI, which further contributes to their higher dropout rate. Given the higher demands to fulfill household and caregiver roles, women may lack the motivation or energy necessary to participate fully in rehabilitation programs[66].

Other factors that should be considered during the recovery period from acute MI include psychosocial stressors, such as limited income and lack of a partner. That women post-MI are likely to be widowed or retired and living on a fixed income may make socioeconomic status (SES) a greater source of stress for women, especially older women, than men. The acknowledged discrepancy in incomes between U.S. males and females and limited access to health insurance following the death of a spouse suggest that SES is a more potent source of stress for women with CAD than men.

Even when women have partners, the partners are often ill or in need of care and unable to offer caregiving assistance. Indeed, widowed, single, or divorced women may be advantaged in not having to worry about the care of a sick spouse. Recovering women may need a chance to discuss the emotional burdens with a nurse practitioner and may also need encouragement to ask others for help. Frasure-Smith demonstrated that an average of 6 hours of emotional and social support provided by a nurse was correlated with a 50% reduction in subsequent deaths following an MI[67].

Caring for women at risk for CAD or recovering from MI is a challenge to the practitioner who must constantly be aware that women may have physiological and psychological needs different from those of men. Searching for treatment methods that are specific to women's health care demands thoughtfulness, surveillance, and perseverance.

—by Paul M. Arnstein, Elizabeth Florentino Buselli,
and Sally H. Rankin

References

1. *U.S. Bureau of the Census: Statistical Abstracts of the United States: 1994* (114th edition). Washington, DC, 1994:95.

2. Wenger NK, Speroff L, Packard B: Cardiovascular health & disease in females. *N Engl J Med* July 22, 1993;329(4):247-56.

3. Kannell WB, Abbott RD: Incidence and prognosis of unrecognized Ml: An update on the Framingham study. *N Engl J Med* 1984;311:1144-47.

4. Selig, PM: The prevention and screening of cardiovascular disease: An update. *Nurs Pract Forum* 1991;2(1):14-18.

5. Lincoff AM, Califf RM, Ellis SG, et al: Thrombolytic therapy for females with MI: Is there a gender gap? *J Am Col Cardiol* 1993;22(7):1780-87.

6. Murdaugh C: Coronary artery disease in women. *J Cardiovasc Nurs* 1994;4(4):35-50.

7. Maynard C, Litwin PE, Marun JS, et al: Gender differences in the treatment and outcome of acute MI. *Arch Intern Med* 1992;152(5):972-76.

8. Steingart RM, Packer M, Hamm P, et al: Sex differences in the management of coronary artery disease. *New Engl J Med* 1991;325:226-30.

9. Kahn SS, Nessim S, Gray R, et al: Increased mortality of women in coronary artery bypass surgery: Evidence of referral bias. *Ann Intern Med* 1990; 1 12:561-67.

10. Berkman LF, Leo-Summers L, Horwitz RL: Emotional support and survival after myocardial infarction. A prospective, population-based study of the elderly. *Ann Intern Med* 1992:117(12):1003-9.

11. Wilkinson P, Ranjadayalaak L, Parsons L, et al: Acute MI in females: survival analysis in the first 6 months. *Br Med J* 1994;309(6954):566-69.

12. Karlson BW, Herlitz J, Hartford M: Prognosis in MI in relation to gender. *Am Heart J* 1994;128(3):477-83.

13. Tsuyuki RT, Teo KK, Ikuta RM, et al: Mortality risk and patterns of practice in 2,070 patients with acute myocardial infarction 1987-1992: Relative importance of age set and medical therapy. *Chest* 1994;105(6):1687-92.

14. Shaw LJ, Miller D, Romeis JC, et al: Gender differences in the noninvasive evaluation and management of patients with

suspected coronary artery disease. *Am Intern Med* 1994;120(7):559-66.

15. Emergency Cardiac Care Committee and Subcommittees, American Heart Association. Guidelines for the cardiopulmonary resuscitation and emergency cardiac care. *JAMA* 1992;268:2175.

16. *U.S. Department of Health Clinical Practice Guideline: Unstable angina: Diagnosis and management.* AHCPR Publication No. 94-0602, May 1994.

17. Pagley PR, Yarzebski J, Goldberg R, et al: Gender differences in the treatment of patients with acute MI. *Arch Intern Med* 1993;625-29.

18. Fiebach NH, Viscoli CM, Hornitz RI: Differences between women and men in survival after myocardial infarction: Biology or methodology? *JAMA* 1990;263(8):1092-96.

19. Keller C, Fleury J, Bergstrom DL: Risk factors for coronary heart disease in African-American women. *Cardiovasc Nurs* 1995;31(2):9-14.

20. Tofler GH, Stone PH, Muller JE, et al: Effects of gender and race on prognosis after myocardial infarction: Adverse prognosis for women, particularly black women. *J Am Coll Cardiol* 1987;9:473.

21. Klatsky AL, Tekawa I, Armstrong MA, et al: The risk of hospitalization for ischemic heart disease among Asian Americans in northern California. *Am J Public Health* 1994;84(10):1672-75.

22. Marenberg ME, Risch N, Berkman LF, et al: Genetic susceptibility to death from coronary heart disease in a study of twins. *N Engl J Med* 1994; 330(15):1041-46.

23. Hunt S, Blickenstaff K, Hopkins PN, et al: Coronary disease risk factors in close relatives of Utah women with early coronary death. *West J Med* 1986;145(3):329-34.

24. Langner NR, Rowe PC, Davies R: The next generation: poor compliance with risk factor guidelines in the children of parents with premature coronary heart disease. *Am J Public Health* 1994;84(1):68-71.

25. Donahue RP, Goldberg RT, Chen Z, et al: The influence of sex and diabetes mellitus on survival following acute myocardial infarction: A community prospective. *J Clinical Epidem* 1993;46(3):245-52.

26. Rich-Edwards JW, Manson JE, Hennekens CH, et al: The primary prevention of coronary heart disease in women. *N Engl J Med* 1995;332(26)175866.

27. Wilson PWF, Garrison RJ, Castelli WP: Postmenopausal estrogen use, cigarette smoking & cardiovascular morbidity in women over 50. The Framingham study. *N Engl J Med* 1985;313:1038-43.

28. Wing RR, Matthews KA, Kuller LH, et al: Waist to hip ratio in middle aged women. Associations with behavioral and psychosocial factors and changes in cardiovascular risk factors. *Arteriosclerosis & Thrombosis* 1991;11(5)125057.

29. Sherman SE, D'Agostino RB, Cobb JL, et al: Physical activity and mortality in females in the Framingham Heart Study. *Am Heart J* 1994;128:879-84.

30. Hawkins RI: Smoking platelets and thrombosis. *Nature* 1972;236:450-52.

31. Willet W, Hennekens CH, Castelli W, et al: Effects of cigarette smoking on fasting triglycerides total cholesterol, HDL, and cholesterol in women. *Am Heart J* 1983;105:4i7-21.

32. Holme I: An analysis of randomized trials evaluating the effect of cholesterol reduction on total mortality and coronary heart disease incidence. *Circulation* 1990;82:1916-24.

33. Miller VT: Lipids, lipoproteins women and cardiovascular disease. *Atherosclerosis* 1994;1 08(supp):S73-82.

34. Castelli WP: A triglyceride issue: A view from Framingham. *Am Heart J* 1986;112:432-37.

35. Notelovitz M, Feldman EB, Gillespy M, et al: Lipid and lipoprotein change in women taking low dose, triphasic oral contraceptives: A controlled comparative 12 month clinical trial. *Am J Obstet Gyn* 1989;160:1269-80.

36. Stampfer M, Colditz G, Willet W, et al: Post menopausal estrogen therapy and cardiovascular disease. *N Engl J Med* 1991;325:756-62.

37. Mason JE: Postmenopausal hormone therapy and atherosclerotic disease. *Am Heart J* 1994;128:1337-43.

38. Psaty BM, Heckbert SR, Atkins D, et al: The risk of myocardial infarction associated with the combined use of estrogens and progestins in postmenopausal women. *Arch Intern Med* 1994;154(12):1333-39.

39. PEPI Trial writing group: Effects of estrogen/progestin regimens on heart disease risk factors in postmenopausal women. The Postmenopausal Estrogen/Progestin Interventions (PEPI) Trial. *JAMA* 1995;273(3):199-208.

40. Amsterdam EA, Hyson D, Kappagoda CT: Nonpharmacologic therapy for coronary artery atherosclerosis: Result of primary and secondary prevention trials. *Am Heart J* 1994;128:1344-52.

41. Lokey EA, Tran ZV: Effect of exercise training on serum tepid and lipoprotein concentrations in women: A meta-analysis. *Int J Sports Med* 1989;10:424-29.

42. Cochrane BL: Acute myocardial infarction in women. *Crit Care Clin North Am* 1992; 4(2):279-89.

43. Bell MR, Holmes DR Jr, Berger PB, et al: The changing in hospital mortality rates of women undergoing percutaneous transluminal coronary angiopiasty. *JAMA* 1993;269(16):2091-95.

44. Haynes SG, Feinleib M: Women, work and coronary heart disease. *Am J Public Health* 1980;70:133-40.

45. La Rosa JH: Women, work and health: Employment as a risk factor for coronary heart disease. *Am J Obstet Gyn* 1988;158:1597-1602.

46. Theorell T: Psychosocial cardiovascular risks on the double loads in women. *Psychother Psychosom* 1991;55:81-89.

47. Keil JE, Loadholt CB, Weinrich MC, et al: Incidence of coronary heart disease in blacks in Charleston, South Carolina. *Am Heart J* 1984;108:779.

48. Wenger NK: Coronary heart disease: Diagnostic decision making. In: Douglas P, ed. *Cardiovascular Health and Disease in Women*. Philadelphia: W.B. Saunders, 1993:22-42.

49. Selzer A, Langston M, Ruggeroli C: Clinical syndrome of variant angina with normal coronary arteriogram. *N Engl J Med* 1976;295:1343.

50. Hendel RC: Myocardial infarction in women. *Cardiology* 1990;77(supp 2):4157.

51. Frasure-Smith N, Lesperance F, Talajic M: Depression and 18 months prognosis after myocardial infarction. *Circulation* 1995;91:999-1005.

52. Williams RB: Prognostic importance of social and economic resources among medically treated patients with angiographically documented CAD. *JAMA* 1992;267(4):520-24.

53. Friedman MM: Stressor and perceived stress in older females with heart disease. *Cardiovasc Nurs* 1993;29(4):25-29.

54. Rankin SH: Going it alone: Female managing recovery from acute MI. *Fam Community Health* 1995;17(4):50-62.

55. Moser DK, Dracup K: Gender differences in treatment-seeking delay in acute myocardial infarction. *Prog Cardiovasc Nurs* 1993;8(1):6-12.

56. Smith, MA, Johnson DG: Evaluation & management of coronary artery disease: Guidelines for the primary care nurse practitioner. *Nurs Pract Forum* 1993;2(1):14-26.

57. Bennett AF, Save HC: Special considerations in cardiovascular assessment of the aged. *Nurs Pract Forum* 1991;2(1):55-60.

58. Dubin S: The physiologic changes of aging. *Orthopedic Nurs* 1992;11(3):45

59. Mukerji V, Holman AJ, Alport MA: The clinical description of angina pectoris in the elderly *Am Heart* 1989;117:705.

60. Klapholz M, Buttrick P: Myocardial function and cardiomyopathy. In Douglas P, ed. *Cardiovascular Health and Disease in Women*. Philadelphia: W.B. Saunders, 1993:105-6.

61. Grays H: *Anatomy: Descriptive and Surgical, 5th ed.* New York: Bounty Books, 1977.

62. de Groot J, Chusid JG: *Correlative Neuroanatomy*, 21st ed. Norwalk: Appleton & Lange, 1991:195-200.

63. Craddock LD: Physical Signs of acute myocardial events. *Emerg Med* 1991;8(15):23-37.

64. Moss AJ, Carleen E, and the Multi-center Postinfarction Research Group: Gender differences in the mortality risk associated with ventricular arrhythmias after myocardial infarction. In: Eaker ED, Packard B, Wenger NK, et al, eds. *Coronary Heart Disease in Women.* New York: Haymarket Doyma 1987:204.

65. Tobin JN, Wassertheil-Smoller S, Wexler JP: Sex bias in considering coronary bypass surgery. *Ann Intern Med* 1987;107: 19-25.

66. Hamilton GA, Seidman RN: A comparison of the recovery period for women and men after an acute myocardial infarction. *Heart Lung* 1993;22(4):308-15.

67. Frasure-Smith N: Long-term follow-up of ischemic heart disease: Life-style monitoring program. *Psychosom Med* 1991;51: 485-512.

Acknowledgments

This project was supported in part by the Boston College University Fellowship Program and a National Institute of Nursing Research Grant R55 NR02617. The authors wish to thank Ann Rolfe for her assistance with an early draft of this manuscript.

Paul M. Arnstein, RN,CS, NP-C, MS, is a family nurse practitioner and a doctoral student at Boston College School of Nursing in Massachusetts.

Elizabeth Florentino Buselli, RN,C, MS, is an adult nurse practitioner doctoral student at Boston College School of Nursing.

Sally H. Rankin, RN, C-NP, PhD, FAAN, is a family nurse practitioner and an associate professor, Nursing, at Boston College School of Nursing.

Chapter 23

Chest Pain with Normal Coronary Arteries

About 20% of patients with chest pain and treadmill evidence of myocardial ischemia have coronary arteries that look normal at angiography. What does this mean? Is more testing necessary? Is treatment appropriate?

Myocardial ischemia and infarction are some of the most significant medical problems faced by physicians and patients in this country. Accordingly, when a patient complains of chest pain, especially chest pain that might be angina pectoris, a noninvasive evaluation is often ordered, usually a treadmill exercise test. If the treadmill ECG is positive—ST segment changes develop during exercise and are consistent with ischemia—most cardiologists order coronary arteriography to confirm the presence and extent of coronary artery disease (CAD).

However, 20% or more of patients with chest pain and abnormal stress test results have normal-appearing coronary arteries at cardiac catheterization. In the 1970s, the unexplained findings of chest pain, stress ECG evidence of myocardial ischemia, and normal coronary anatomy were dubbed syndrome X (not to be confused with the other, metabolic, syndrome X—the complex that includes hypertension, hypertriglyceridemia, and glucose intolerance). While the term syndrome X is still sometimes used to describe this rather baffling

"Chest Pain with Normal Coronary Arteries," by Ezra A. Amsterdam, Mark Apfelbaum, Richard O. Cannon III, and Gary Hoff, in *Patient Care*, March 15, 1997, Vol. 31, No. 5, Pg. 43(7), © 1997 Medical Economics Publishing; reprinted with permission.

cardiac phenomenon, it has fallen out of favor because these patients are heterogeneous in their clinical presentation, pathophysiology, and management. They may or may not have objective, reproducible evidence of myocardial ischemia, and the condition remains a challenging clinical problem.

The Puzzle

Patients with this problem are usually female and report chest discomfort or pain that resembles angina pectoris, although the pain is more often atypical. Their response to exercise treadmill testing may be similar to that of patients with ischemic heart disease, including reproduction of the chest pain and significant ST segment depression, although some patients have no pain, only ST segment changes. Cardiac catheterization, however, reveals normal or nearly normal coronary arteries.

Theories advanced to explain why many patients with apparently normal coronary arteries display signs consistent with myocardial ischemia have been highly contentious. Some authorities have suggested that the pain is caused by real—but undetectable—ischemia. Others say it occurs as a result of disease in other organs such as the stomach or esophagus, or that it is a psychiatric problem. Still others believe the pain is a manifestation of a heart that is more sensitive than others to certain kinds of stimuli. No consensus yet exists, but at least some of the puzzle is becoming clearer.

Is Microvascular Pathology at Fault?

Several years ago, the term "microvascular angina" was coined to explain the condition that had been called syndrome X.[1] Since pathologic changes had not been demonstrated in epicardial coronary arteries despite findings suggesting ischemia, the possibility of microvascular pathology was intriguing. The microvascular angina model proposes that patients with angina-like chest pain, abnormal stress ECG findings, and normal epicardial coronary arteries have patchy areas (or perhaps even large segments) of myocardium with reduced blood flow caused by abnormal microvascular function.[2]

Researchers have attempted for more than 20 years to uncover objective evidence of myocardial ischemia during episodes of chest pain in these patients. However, invasive hemodynamic studies, including measurement of lactate in the coronary sinus, determination of pulmonary artery pressures during stress testing, and measurement of coronary oxygen saturations, among others, have failed to provide convincing evidence of ischemia. Nonetheless, the majority of patients with chest pain and normal or nearly normal coronary arteries probably do not have microvascular dysfunction. It's long been noted that even though the ECG appears abnormal during rapid atrial pacing, cardiac output response and other hemodynamic measures of left ventricular function differ considerably between patients with documented CAD and those with chest pain and normal coronary arteries. In addition, the long-term survival of patients with chest pain and normal coronary arteries is excellent, which in itself speaks against significant myocardial ischemia.

Patchy myocardial ischemia may be present in areas too small to cause a significant reduction in myocardial function, or a reduction in wall motion may be too tiny to be detected by current methods. The evidence for ischemia in the majority of these patients, however, remains sketchy at best.

A Sensitive Heart?

Researchers at the National Institutes of Health have postulated that many of these patients simply have heightened pain perception, so-called sensitive hearts.[3] In one study of 36 patients with chest pain and normal coronary arteries, pacing the heart at a rate only 5 beats per minute (bpm) faster than resting rates induced the characteristic chest pain in 86%.[4] In addition, chest pain was also provoked in 56% of the same group during injection of contrast material into the left coronary artery. These findings are supported by other investigators who provoked chest pain in a similar group of patients by moving a catheter within the right ventricle or right atrium; in comparison, this maneuver failed to cause pain in most patients with documented mitral valve disease or CAD.[5]

The exact mechanism of enhanced pain sensitivity in patients with sensitive hearts is unknown. Exaggerated visceral sensitivity, perhaps mediated by adenosine or other naturally occurring metabolic products, may be at fault.

Overall, the etiology of chest pain in patients with normal coronary arteries remains unclear, and several mechanisms may be involved. According to some experts, an area that requires further elucidation is the role of abnormal coronary vasodilator reserve, as well as its association with hypertrophy of the left ventricle. With contemporary interest in the vascular endothelium, such information is likely to be forthcoming and may lead to specific therapeutic approaches to enhance coronary vasodilator reserve. These were among the topics discussed at a recent workshop on coronary microcirculation held at the National Heart, Lung, and Blood Institute (NHLBI).[6] Only a small proportion of these patients are likely to have microvascular angina. Many, if not most, probably have sensitive hearts that overreact to small-scale stimuli that have no effect on normal or even ischemic myocardium. Moreover, a number of other possibilities deserve consideration in any patient with chest pain, including GI, musculoskeletal, and psychiatric conditions.

Diagnosing Chest Pain

When patients present with chest pain, a careful exploration of the history, especially of the chest pain itself, is crucial.

- What is the quality of the chest discomfort? Its location? Does it radiate? Does pain occur with swallowing? Is there a sensation of something stuck in the throat?

- Is the patient aware of factors that cause or relieve the pain?

- How long does an episode typically last?

- Are other symptoms present with the pain?

- Is the discomfort reproducible with similar levels of exertion?

- How long ago did the episodes of pain start?

The answers to these questions help determine whether the patient's chest discomfort is typical or atypical of angina pectoris.

Determining the patient's cardiovascular risk profile allows you to estimate the probability of coronary disease. Hypertension, hyperlipidemia, cigarette smoking, diabetes mellitus, and obesity increase the likelihood of CAD. Other factors make the diagnosis of CAD less likely. The prevalence of coronary disease in premenopausal women, for example, is exceedingly low. The situation is reversed among older patients with several risk factors and typical angina pectoris.

Treadmill Testing and Catheterization

Depending on your assessment of the history, the next step is usually exercise treadmill testing. In many patients, the additional predictive power of imaging is not needed. In those with a high probability of CAD, however, many cardiologists add either myocardial scintigraphy or two-dimensional echocardiography to delineate specific areas of reduced myocardial function and, hence, reduced perfusion.

If the patient's risk of CAD is low, the need for myocardial imaging during cardiac stress testing is unclear since imaging adds little to posttest predictive power. Stress ECGs alone are clearly more cost-effective in such patients.

If stress testing suggests ischemia, many clinicians assume that cardiac catheterization is the next essential step, but this is not always the case. The prevalence of coronary disease in premenopausal women with typical chest pain is probably around 1%. If the treadmill test is positive, given a sensitivity and specificity for stress ECGs of approximately 60% and 90%, respectively, the posttest probability that such a woman with a positive test actually has coronary artery disease is only 6%. Conversely, a woman in this group with a negative test has a 99% probability of having normal coronary arteries. In short, a stress test is no more reliable for ruling out myocardial ischemia than the history and physical examination are. In such patients, conservative management and watchful expectancy make costly, invasive procedures such as coronary arteriography unnecessary.

The Role of Perfusion Imaging

For patients at higher risk for CAD, however, myocardial perfusion imaging may be necessary. Although coronary anglograms may be normal in appearance, the possibility of myocardial ischemia still exists. In at least one study, anglographic images of coronary arteries in patients with chest pain and abnormal stress ECGs appeared normal, but intravascular ultrasound showed abnormal intimal thickening or atheromatous plaque in 18 of 30 patients.[7] Seventeen of these 18 patients also had abnormal results on thallium or stress echocardiography. Of the 12 patients with normal findings by intravascular ultrasound, only two had abnormal stress imaging studies.

In contrast, if stress perfusion imaging is normal, the patient is unlikely to have clinically significant CAD. The prognosis is excellent in these patients, and further cardiovascular evaluation is probably unnecessary. Depending on the history and the nature of the symptoms, consider another diagnosis. A substantial number of people with angina—like pain have an esophageal motility disorder.[8] Gastroesophageal reflux is another possibility. Finally, several psychiatric disorders may cause symptoms that mimic angina pectoris, especially panic disorder and generalized anxiety disorder.[9]

Selecting an Appropriate Management Strategy

Treating patients with chronic pain is notoriously difficult, and those with chest pain and normal coronary arteries are no exception. When a patient with an abnormal stress test is found to have apparently normal coronary arteries, the first and most important step is to reassure the patient that the prognosis is excellent. Don't underestimate the importance of this seemingly simple step, especially since no other treatment is widely used or universally accepted.

Even with this reassurance, chest pain often continues to be a problem for many patients. Some continue to limit their activities. Moreover, many people describe their pain as either unchanged or worse after a negative work-up. A substantial minority may continue to believe that they have heart disease despite the physician's careful explanation of the normal findings and excellent prognosis.

Trials of antianginal medications, including nitrates, [Beta]-blockers, and calcium channel blockers, have been used with little success in patients with chest pain and normal coronary arteries. Some investigators have reported success with long-acting nitrates, although the patients studied had normal coronary anglograms and either coronary intimal thickening or atherosclerotic plaque detected by intravascular ultrasound. Recent reports have also shown some benefit associated with angiotensin-converting enzyme inhibitors, specifically enalapril maleate.(*)[10,11]

For the majority of patients with chest pain with normal coronary arteries, treatment remains problematic. For those with proven or possible gastroesophageal reflux, a trial of omeprazole, 20 mg daily, may be worthwhile. Patients with panic disorder may respond to psychotherapy, counseling, a benzodiazepine, or an antidepressant. For a large percentage of patients with chest pain despite normal coronary anglograms, imipramine HCI, 50 mg nightly, reduces symptoms, regardless of whether patients have evidence of cardiac sensitivity, esophageal disease, or a psychiatric disorder.[12]

(*) Unlabeled use.

References

1. Cannon RO III, Epstein SE: "Microvascular angina" as a cause of chest pain with angiographically normal coronary arteries, editorial. *Am J Cardiol* 1988; 61:1338-1343.

2. Cannon RO III: Microvascular angina: Cardiovascular investigations regarding pathophysiology and management, *Med Clin North Am* 1991; 75:1097-1118.

3. Cannon RO III: The sensitive heart: A syndrome of abnormal cardiac pain perception. *JAMA* 1995; 273:883-887.

4. Cannon RO III, Quyyumi AA, Schenke WH, et al: Abnormal cardiac sensitivity in patients with chest pain and normal coronary arteries. *J Am Coll Cardiol* 1990;16:1359-1366.

5. Chauhan A, Mullins PA, Thuraisingham SI, et al: Abnormal cardiac pain perception in syndrome X. *J Am Coll Cardiol* 1994; 24:329-335.

6. Chillon WM: Coronary microcirculation in health and disease: Summary of an NHLBI workshop. *Circulation* 1997; 95:522-528.

7. Wiederman JG, Schwartz A, Apfelbaum M: Anatomic and physiologic heterogeneity in patients with syndrome X: An intravascular ultrasound study. *J Am Coll* Cardiol 1995; 25:1310-1317.

8. Richter JE, Bradley LA, Castell DO: Esophageal chest pain: Current controversies in pathogenesis, diagnosis, and therapy. *Ann Intern Med* 1989; 110:66-78.

9. Beitmen BD, Vaskar M, Lamperti JW, et al: Panic; disorder in patients with chest pain and angiographically normal coronary arteries. *Am J Cardiol* 1989; 63:1399-1403.

10. Kaski JC, Rosano G, Gavrielides S, et al: Effects of angiotensin-converting enzyme inhibition on exercise-induced angina and ST segment depression in patients with microvascular angina. *J Am Coll Cardiol* 1994; 23:652-657.

11. Iriarte MM, Caso R, Murga N, at al: Microvascular angina in systemic hypertension: Diagnosis and treatment with enalapril. *Am J Cardiol* 1995; 76:31 D-34D.

12. Cannon RO III, Quyyumi AA, Mincemoyer R, et al: Imipramine in patients with chest pain despite normal coronary angiograms. *N Engl J Med* 1994; 330:1411-1417

Suggested Reading

Botker HE, Mailer N, Oyesen P, et al: Insulin Resistance in Microvascular Angina (Syndrome X). *Lancet* 1993; 342:136-140.

Egashira K, Hirooka Y, Kuga T, et al: Effects of L-arginine supplementation on endothelium-dependent coronary vasodilation in patients with angina pectoris and normal coronary arteriograms, *Circulation* 1996; 94:130-134.

Egashira K, Inou T, Hirooka Y, et al: Evidence of impaired endothelium-dependent coronary vasodilation in patients with angina pectoris and normal coronary angiograms. *N Engl J Med* 1993; 328:1659-1664.

Iriarte M, Caso R, Murga N, et al: Microvascular angina pectoris in hypertensive patients with left ventricular hypertrophy and diagnostic value of exercise thallium201 scintigraphy. *Am J Cardiol* 1995; 75:335-339.

Kaski JC, Elliott PM: Angina pectoris and normal coronary arteriograms: Clinical presentation and hemodynamic characteristics. *Am J Cardiol* 1995; 76:35D-42D.

Zhang Y, Jeffery S, Badey J, et al: Angiotensin-converting enzyme insertion/deletion polymorphism in angina pectoris with normal coronary arteriograms. *Am J Cardiol* 1996; 77:877-879.

Using Bayes' Theorem to Understand Test Results

If the prevalence of a disease in a given population is known, and if the sensitivity and specificity of the test being ordered are also known, the predictive value of a positive test—the likelihood that the patient actually has the disease—can be calculated. This is the essence of Bayes' theorem.

The possibility of coronary artery disease (CAD) in a patient is related to the person's age, gender, type of pain, and the presence or absence of risk factors such as hyperlipidemia, hypertension, cigarette smoking, family history, diabetes mellitus, and obesity, among others. A premenopausal woman without risk factors, even with typical angina pectoris, belongs to a population in which the prevalence of CAD is only 1%. On the other hand, a man 60 or older with typical angina and several risk factors for cardiovascular disease belongs to a group of patients in which the probability of CAD is as high as 90%.

An exercise treadmill test has sensitivity—true-positives divided by the sum of true-positives and false-negatives—of about 60% and specificity—true-negatives divided by the sum of true-negatives and false-positives—of about 90%. If a treadmill test is ordered, the positive posttest predictive power is only 6% for the premenopausal woman, but 75% for the man older than 60. The negative posttest predictive power for the two patients in question is 99% and 11%, respectively.

So a negative test result for the woman doesn't help rule out CAD because the negative posttest predictive power is identical to that of the history and physical alone. Moreover, a positive test for her adds very little positive predictive power. In the high-risk, older male, a negative test actually has less posttest predictive power than the history and physical, as does a positive test. Thus, neither patient described here would necessarily benefit from treadmill testing in these circumstances because the test does not add significantly to predictive power.

Suppose a patient falls into an intermediate group with a 50% prevalence of coronary disease—perhaps a man younger than 40 with strong family history and typical angina pectoris. Again assuming that a treadmill test has a sensitivity of about 60% and a specificity of 90%, a positive treadmill test has a posttest positive predictive power of 86% and a negative predictive power of 69%. Therefore, treadmill testing is quite useful in this intermediate-risk group because the results add substantially to the pretest findings.

Remember that the exercise test may provide additional information beyond the conventional dichotomous positive or negative result. For example, a positive test occurring at a low workload and low heart rate—120 beats per minute (bpm) or less—accompanied by an ST segment depression of more than 2 mm is far more likely to suggest high risk for CAD than an ST segment elevation of 1 mm at a high workload and heart rate (150 bpm or more). The latter is either a false-positive or a low-risk, true-positive. The former is a high-risk, true-positive with a high probability of CAD.

Article Consultants

Ezra A. Amsterdam, MD, is Professor of Medicine (Cardiology), University of California, Davis, School of Medicine; and Director, Cardiac Care Unit, University of California, Davis Medical Center, Sacramento. He is a member of the Patient Care Subspecialist Advisory Board.

Mark Apfelbaum, MD, is Associate Director, Interventional Cardiology Center, Columbia-Presbyterian Medical Center, New York City.

Richard O. Cannon III, MD, is Deputy Chief for Clinical Services, Cardiology Branch, National Heart, Lung, and Blood Institute, National Institutes of Health, Bethesda, Md.

Chapter 24

Outlook for Women after Bypass Surgery

Several studies have shown higher rates of mortality for women who have coronary artery disease treated with bypass surgery or angioplasty.

Theories abound on why women may have worse outcomes than men. Among them is the observation that women have smaller blood vessels and are older when coronary disease finally develops and is diagnosed. Some critics of the health-care system suggest that the higher mortality for women may be due to insensitivity to women's symptoms on the part of physicians, leading to later recognition of coronary disease.

Recent research raises the question, however, of whether this "gender gap" exists at all. In this study, researchers analyzed data from 1,829 patients who were enrolled in the Bypass Angioplasty Revascularization Investigation (BARI) study. This study enrolled men and women with symptoms due to coronary disease in two or more vessels and randomly assigned them to percutaneous transluminal coronary angioplasty (PTCA) or coronary artery bypass graft surgery (CABG). Women constituted 27% of the study population.

At 5.4 years of follow-up, about the same percentage of women and men had died—13% and 12%, respectively. However, researchers noted that the women in the study were older and were more likely to have several factors that would be expected to increase their chances of dying—including congestive heart failure, high blood pressure, diabetes, and unstable angina. After using statistical techniques to adjust for these differences, the researchers concluded that women actually had a 40% lower risk of death than men did. (*Circulation*, Vol. 98, No. 13, pp. 1279-1285.)

These findings provide encouragement that women may not truly be at increased risk for dying after bypass surgery or angioplasty. This study suggests that the basic treatment strategies for men and women with coronary disease should be similar. However, the data also show that women tend to be older when they develop the need for angioplasty or surgery and are more likely to have important risk factors for subsequent complications.

Part Four

The Hormone Replacement Therapy Controversy

Chapter 25

Hormone Replacement Therapy and Heart Disease: The PEPI Trial

Heart disease is the leading cause of death and illness for American women. Each year, about 250,000 American women die of coronary heart disease, the main form of heart disease. And nearly 90,000 die each year of stroke.

Heart disease is also the leading cause of death for men, but men and women differ in how and when heart disease develops. Typically, heart disease develops about 10 years later in women than in men.

The reason for this may be tied to women's production of the hormone estrogen. When women go through menopause, their ovaries essentially stop making estrogen and their risk of heart disease rises dramatically. Eventually, it nearly equals that of men.

What Is Hormone Replacement Therapy?

Menopause denotes the completion of a full year without a period, including any bleeding, even spotting. It usually happens between the ages of 45 and 54.

Menopause can occur naturally or as the result of surgery. The procedure, called a hysterectomy, removes the uterus and sometimes the ovaries and fallopian tubes as well. Although a woman no longer has periods after a hysterectomy, she does not go through menopause unless both ovaries are removed—otherwise, menopause still occurs naturally.

National Heart, Lung, and Blood Institute (NHLBI), NIH Publication No. 95-3277, August 1995.

191

Whether menopause occurs naturally or surgically, many women experience symptoms as their body adjusts to the fall in estrogen. The most common symptoms are hot flashes and flushes, sweats, and sleep disturbances. Other changes occur that may produce no recognized symptoms, such as an increased rate of bone loss that may result in osteoporosis. The osteoporosis may, in turn, lead to bone fractures usually after age 70.

These symptoms may interfere with a woman's regular activities. To relieve the symptoms, doctors may prescribe "hormone replacement therapy" (HRT). Today, this term is used to describe treatment with either estrogen alone or with estrogen and another hormone called progestin. The two hormones help regulate a woman's menstrual cycle and progestin is added to prevent the overgrowth (or hyperplasia) of cells in the lining of the uterus.

Hormone therapy goes by various names, depending on the hormones used. "Estrogen replacement therapy" refers to treatment that uses only estrogen. "Combined progestin/estrogen replacement therapy" (PERT) is the use of both hormones.

Replacement therapies can be taken in several ways, including orally or through a patch on the skin. The hormones may be taken daily or on only certain days of the month.

Table 25.1. The Top Five Causes of Death for American Women in 1992 Were:

• Heart disease	360,000
• Cancer (all types)	246,000
Select types	
Lung	56,000
Breast	43,000
Ovarian	12,000
Cervical	5,000
Endometrial	3,000
• Stroke	87,000
• Chronic obstructive pulmonary disease	41,000
• Pneumonia/influenza	40,000

1989 data, most recent available

New Possibilities for HRT

Women can greatly reduce their chance of developing heart disease by following certain behaviors—eating low-saturated fat, low-cholesterol foods; not smoking; being physically active; and keeping a healthy weight.

But, if estrogen helps protect women against heart disease, then it might offer another valuable preventive measure for many women past menopause.

Through the years, evidence has accumulated suggesting that estrogen acts on some of the factors that define a woman's risk of heart disease. For instance, estrogen seems to affect the levels in the blood of two important lipoproteins-high-density lipoprotein (HDL) and low-density lipoprotein (LDL). High-density lipoprotein helps remove cholesterol from the blood and is called the "good" cholesterol. Low-density lipoprotein carries most of the cholesterol and fat through blood vessels, where it can build up. LDL is called the "bad" cholesterol.

Both HDL and LDL are important risk factors for heart disease. For women, a low level of HDL appears to be the better predictor of heart disease risk—for men, a high LDL appears to be the better predictor. Estrogen seems to increase HDL and decrease LDL.

But it was thought that in addition to its benefits, estrogen use also posed risks—such as increasing both blood pressure and the chance of cancer of the endometrium, the lining of the uterus. The increased risk of endometrial cancer associated with estrogen-only therapy seems to be eliminated when estrogen is given with progestin. However, it was not known whether combined therapy might negate estrogen's beneficial effects on heart disease risk factors and bone loss.

The PEPI Study

To learn more about estrogen's possible benefits and risks, the National Heart, Lung, and Blood Institute (NHLBI) and other units of the National Institutes of Health started a major clinical trial in 1987—the "Postmenopausal Estrogen/Progestin Interventions Trial," called PEPI.

PEPI's other sponsors are the National Institute of Child Health and Human Development, the National Institute of Arthritis and Musculoskeletal and Skin Diseases, the National Institute of Diabetes and Digestive and Kidney Diseases, and the National Institute on Aging.

PEPI was conducted at seven clinical centers across the United States. It followed 875 women, ages 45-64, for 3 years. All were healthy and postmenopausal, and about a third had had a hysterectomy. Participants included a variety of races but were predominantly white.

The women were closely monitored and had such tests as a yearly physical examination, mammogram, and, for those with a uterus, an endometrial biopsy.

The main goal was to see what effects different hormone regimens would have on some key risk factors for heart disease. The study also collected other information, including the regimens' effects on quality of life, bone mass, and the risk of endometrial changes that might progress into cancer.

The four hormone regimens tested were:

- Estrogen alone, taken daily
- Estrogen taken daily and a synthetic progestin (medroxyprogesterone acetate), taken 12 days a month
- Estrogen and synthetic progestin taken daily
- Estrogen taken daily plus a natural progesterone (micronized progesterone), taken 12 days a month

The effects of these regimens were compared with those of a placebo, a substance that looks like the real drug but has no biologic effect. The trial also compared for the first time the effects of cyclic and continuous use of progestin. Cyclic use means taking a medication for only some days of each month, while continuous use means taking the drug daily throughout the month. A main reason for the comparison was to see if continuous use produced less bleeding.

First Results—Heart Disease Risk Factors

A huge amount of information was collected in PEPI. Thus, the results will take time to be fully analyzed. But, because of their importance to women and their doctors, the findings are being released as they become available. The first results, reported here, cover PEPI's findings on changes in heart disease risk factors and on hormone safety.

For heart disease risk factors, key results are:

- Estrogen-only therapy raises the level of good HDL cholesterol. (This finding had been previously reported in short-term studies and can now be expanded to long-term effects.)

- The combined estrogen-progestin therapies also increased HDL levels, although less than estrogen alone. At the same time, the addition of progestin produced the desired effect of reducing the increased risk of overgrowth of the lining of the uterus (endometrial hyperplasia) associated with estrogen-only therapy. The natural micronized progesterone produced a higher HDL level than the synthetic form.

- All of the hormone regimens decreased the level of the "bad" LDL cholesterol about equally well.

- Blood pressure was not increased by any of the hormone regimens.

- Fibrinogen levels were decreased by all of the hormones, which is thought to be a desirable change. Fibrinogen allows clots to form more readily, which increases the risk of heart disease and stroke.

- Insulin levels were not significantly affected by any of the hormone regimens. While fasting blood glucose seemed to be reduced by all of the regimens, the blood glucose 2 hours after eating seemed to be elevated by varying degrees. The importance of these changes is unclear, but they are of interest because of their relationship to carbohydrate metabolism and potentially to diabetes, which would in turn affect the risk of heart disease. These altered glucose levels need further evaluation.

- All of the hormone regimens caused a rise in triglyceride levels. These are fatty substances carried through the blood to tissues, where they are stored for use as energy. Their link to heart disease risk is not clear.

- None of the hormone regimens caused a significant weight gain.

For hormone safety, a key result is:

- Women with a uterus who took only estrogen had a higher risk of changes to the uterus lining. A third of these women developed serious abnormal cell growth of the endometrium. These hyperplasias can become cancerous but, if caught early, are treatable.

PEPI did not last long enough to study the effect of hormone therapy on the risk of breast cancer.

Table 25.2 Hormone Therapy with Estrogen does Not:

- Increase blood pressure
- Put women with high blood pressure at even greater risk of heart disease
- Cause weight gain

What Do PEPI's Results Mean for You?

These results give women and their doctors guidelines to use in considering postmenopausal hormone therapy. The results show that hormone therapy can benefit heart disease risk factors. They also emphasize that the choice of a hormone regimen must be based on many factors, including, a woman's heart disease risk profile.

Women need to be involved in decisions about their health care. In deciding whether to use a postmenopausal hormone regimen, women should consider these guidelines:

- Postmenopausal women who have not had a hysterectomy should consider taking a combination therapy that uses estrogen and progestin. If a woman with a uterus takes estrogen alone, she should have a yearly endometrial biopsy because of the risk of serious hyperplasias—this is vital for good health.

- Postmenopausal women who have had a hysterectomy should consider taking estrogen alone. These women are at no risk of endometrial changes, since they no longer have a uterus.

Will You Need Follow-up Tests?

Every woman should watch her health and this means taking a preventive approach.

For instance, women should be alert for side effects from any treatment, including hormone therapy. Women should discuss any side effect with their doctor.

If a woman has a uterus and takes estrogen-only therapy, she should have a yearly endometrial biopsy.

Finally, all women should know their cholesterol number—those for total, HDL, and LDL. If these numbers are known and are all right, then the levels can be remeasured within 5 years.

If women do not know these numbers, then they should have their total, HDL, and LDL cholesterol levels measured before starting a hormone regimen. If the decision to use replacement therapy is related to an expected improvement in HDL and LDL levels, then having this information at the outset gives "baseline measures" against which later tests can be compared. The response to hormone replacement can be measured in 6 or 12 months, or as advised by the doctor. If the levels are acceptable at that time, then they can be measured again once every 5 years. Those with high LDL cholesterol will have to take further steps to lower it.

What Lies Ahead?

PEPI is expected to release more findings in the future on endometrial and bone mass changes, and the effects of hormone therapies on quality of life.

Although data from PEPI trial address a number of important issues, they will not answer all of the questions about the effects of replacement therapies. For instance, remaining questions include: How long should hormone therapy be taken? What's the best age for a woman to start a hormone regimen? Do hormones actually reduce heart attacks and strokes?

Uncertainties also remain about the effects of hormone replacement therapies on breast cancer risk. So far, studies have reported conflicting findings. Most have reported a modest or no increased risk. However, others have reported significant increased risk in long-term hormone replacement users. Additional research is needed to more accurately assess whether there is an increased breast cancer risk and, if so, how to weigh this risk with the benefits related to hormone replacement use. Evidence currently available suggests that there is a small increased risk of breast cancer in hormone replacement users but that, for most women, the benefits of therapy probably outweigh the risks. Studies now under way include a large clinical trial and should eventually provide a basis for the development of more definitive guidelines.

Researchers at the National Institutes of Health and elsewhere are studying these and other questions about the effects of hormone replacement therapies.

Talking with Your Doctor

Women need to be involved in their health care. Talk to your doctor about whether you should take a postmenopausal hormone therapy. Ask questions and express your concerns. For example:

- Should I take hormones? Why?
- How could hormone therapy improve my heart disease risk factor profile?
- At what age should I begin?
- What is the best regimen for me? Why?
- How long should I stay on the therapy?
- If breast cancer has occurred in my family, should I consider HRT?
- If I have had breast cancer, should I consider HRT?
- What follow up tests will I need? How often mill I need to have each test?

Your risk profile may change over time—review your health status with your doctor regularly.

Your Heart Disease Risk Profile

Certain factors can increase your chance of developing heart disease. These are called "risk factors. "

The more risk factors you have, the more likely you are to develop heart disease and the risk multiplies with each additional risk factor. So it is important to have as few risk factors as possible.

Some risk factors are beyond your control; others can be modified to reduce your heart disease risk. You can reduce your risk by adopting a healthier lifestyle—and, as a bonus, you'll look and feel better too.

In choosing a hormone therapy, you and your doctor should talk over your heart disease risk profile.

The major risk factors for heart disease are as follows:

Risk factors beyond your control:

- Being age 55 or older
- Having a family history of early heart disease (this means having a mother or sister who has been diagnosed with heart disease before age 65, or a father or brother diagnosed before age 55)

Risk factors under your control:

- Cigarette smoking

- High blood cholesterol
- High blood pressure
- Diabetes (high blood sugar)
- Obesity
- Physical inactivity

Additional factors to consider:

- If you drink alcohol, do so in moderation. While not a direct heart disease risk factor, drinking too much increases your risk of high blood pressure, which then increases your chance of heart disease. The Dietary Guidelines for Americans recommend that, for overall health, women have no more than one drink a day. A drink would be 1.5 ounces of 80-proof whiskey, 5 ounces of wine, or 12 ounces of beer (regular or light).

- Limit salt and sodium intake. Sodium too is not a direct heart disease risk factor but increases the risk of high blood pressure. Salt is one form of sodium, so you need to watch your use of both. This includes whatever is added during cooking and at the table. Experts advise a total daily salt intake of no more than 6 grams, which equals about 2,400 milligrams of sodium.

For More Information

But, though questions remain, women not wait to reduce their risk of heart disease. NHLBI has information to help women improve their risk profile. Materials cover such topics as heart-healthy eating plans and ways to become physically active.

Contact:

NHLBI Information Center
P.O. Box 30105
Bethesda, MD 20824-0105
Phone: (301) 251-1222

Chapter 26

Estrogen Replacement Therapy—Pros and Cons

Jane Doe is a 53-year-old woman in generally good health. She worries, though, because her blood pressure is high and her cholesterol profile is less than optimum—since her level of the "bad" low-density-lipoprotein (LDL) cholesterol is somewhat elevated and her "good" high-density-lipoprotein (HDL) cholesterol is a bit low. All of these factors place her at an increased risk of coronary artery disease.

She sees a new physician for a checkup and remarks that her mother died of a heart attack at age 59. Jane Doe herself has already quit smoking, lowered the fat in her diet, and started getting some type of exercise at least four times a week, but she wonders what more she can do to reduce her risk of heart disease. Her doctor asks about her menstrual periods, and she responds that she stopped menstruating a year ago. Her physician brings up estrogen-replacement therapy.

A good idea? For this particular woman, the answer is probably yes. But what if Jane Doe's mother had no history of heart disease and had developed breast cancer when she was 45? Estrogen replacement might not be such a good idea for Jane Doe because of her lower probability of having a heart attack and her higher risk of developing breast cancer. So how does someone decide?

Whether or not to take estrogens after menopause is a decision that should depend on a balance between risks and benefits, and this balance

---

Excerpted from the March, 1996 issue of *Harvard Heart Letter*, © 1996 President and Fellows of Harvard College; reprinted with permission.

varies among women. The major benefits of postmenopausal estrogen therapy are reductions in the risk of heart disease and osteoporosis (as well as symptomatic relief from postmenopausal symptoms such as hot flashes and vaginal dryness). The potential risks are increased chances of breast cancer and endometrial cancer (cancer of the uterus)—although the latter risk seems to disappear if the woman takes progesterone along with the estrogen twelve or more days a month. (Progesterone is typically taken in the form of medroxyprogesterone, or Provera.) What follows is the current knowledge about these benefits and risks.

Heart Disease

Though the controversy over whether estrogen-replacement therapy reduces the probability of a heart attack is not completely settled, several epidemiologic studies have demonstrated a significantly reduced risk among women who take it. Among 48,470 postmenopausal participants in the Nurses' Health Study, women taking estrogen-replacement therapy had a risk of coronary artery disease about half that of those not using estrogen, after adjusting for age and other risk factors for coronary artery disease.

Similar conclusions emerged from a "meta-analysis" by Harvard researchers who combined the results of thirty epidemiologic investigations—including prospective studies that followed users and non-users of estrogen replacement to see who developed coronary disease; retrospective studies that looked back at estrogen-use patterns of women who did or did not develop coronary disease; and cross-sectional studies that examined the relationship between estrogen use and the extent of coronary atherosclerosis (cholesterol-laden deposits that line and narrow the interior walls of arteries). In the final analysis, the researchers concluded that estrogen replacement lowered the risk of coronary artery disease by 44%.

These findings are particularly compelling since as many as one-third of all women 65 and older have coronary artery disease, which is by far the leading cause of death in this group. However, it is important to recognize that estimates of reduced heart-disease risk associated with post-menopausal estrogen replacement have come from observational studies—in which researchers looked at disease rates among women who had themselves decided or been advised by their physicians to take estrogen. (The most reliable type of investigation is a randomized study—in which women are randomly assigned to take or not take estrogen after menopause.)

Some experts have speculated that women who use estrogen replacement tend to be healthier in ways that might decrease their heart-disease risk—they may exercise more, eat healthier diets, or see their physicians more often. As a result, it is impossible to say with certainty that it is the estrogen—rather than something else about the women who use this hormone—that accounts for the lower heart-disease risk.

Still, there are a number of biologic reasons why estrogen should be good for the heart. For one, estrogen-replacement therapy is associated with a significant increase in HDL cholesterol and a significant decrease in LDL cholesterol, on the order of 15% each. Second, studies have shown positive effects of estrogen on the reactivity of blood vessels. For example, some women given estrogen (injected into their arteries or administered in a potent oral form) experienced widening (dilatation) of their blood vessels in response to certain stimuli—a phenomenon that might be expected to protect the heart by improving blood flow. Third, estrogen replacement may possibly decrease blood clotting, one of the factors thought to precipitate a heart attack. For example, lower blood levels of fibrinogen, a protein involved in blood clotting, have been reported in estrogen users. Fourth, estrogen replacement may improve the body's response to insulin, as evidenced by lower fasting insulin levels among estrogen users. (Decreased sensitivity to insulin, or "insulin resistance," is another independent risk factor for coronary artery disease.) Finally, some, though not all, studies have reported lower blood pressures in estrogen users than in nonusers.

Most epidemiologic and physiologic studies of hormone replacement and the heart have focused on estrogen therapy alone, and some physicians have been concerned that the combined estrogen/progesterone regimens commonly used to protect against endometrial cancer might not confer the same cardiovascular benefit as estrogen alone. This concern arose because of the observation that Provera (a progestin) might have adverse effects on cholesterol levels, lowering HDL and raising LDL. Recently, results of a study known as the Postmenopausal Estrogen/Progestin Intervention (PEPI) Trial proved reassuring on this point. Women who were assigned to take a combination of estrogen (Premarin) and Provera therapy had reductions in LDL that were similar to those in women on estrogen alone, although the HDL levels were not increased to quite the same extent. Women on combined therapy also had fibrinogen levels comparable to women on estrogen alone, suggesting that progesterone did not block the potential favorable effects of estrogen on blood cougulability.

Osteoporosis

Osteoporosis, thinning of bones that can result from estrogen deficiency at and after menopause, is much less likely to occur among users of post-menopausal estrogen replacement than among nonusers. Estrogen therapy typically arrests bone loss and may even cause small but significant increases in bone density. Since one in six women has a hip fracture during her lifetime, and far more have vertebral fractures, the benefits of estrogen in the prevention and treatment of this problem can be important. Recently, other medications that are not estrogens have become available to treat osteoporosis in women with this condition who should not take the female hormones.

Potential Risks

Endometrial Cancer Postmenopausal women who have a uterus and take estrogen therapy by itself have approximately six times the risk of endometrial cancer as do nonusers. However, the increased risk seems to disappear when progesterone is added to the regimen. A recent study showed that 33% of women who used estrogen alone developed endometrial adenomatous hyperplasia (considered to be a precursor of endometrial cancer), compared with only 1% of women on a combined estrogen-progestin regimen. Thus, the concomitant use of progesterone with estrogen appears to protect against endometrial cancer.

Breast Cancer

The risk of breast cancer associated with postmenopausal estrogen therapy continues to remain controversial. Last summer, two reports received a great deal of media attention. The first, from the Nurses' Health Study, found a significantly increased risk of breast cancer (approximately 40% increase) among women currently taking either estrogen replacement alone or combined estrogen/progestin therapy. Women who had been using hormones longer had higher risks than short-term users, and in fact risks did not rise significantly until after five years of use. Past users were not at increased risk of breast cancer. Relative risks for breast cancer were highest in older women (60-64 years of age), particularly those who had been using hormones for at least five years. Of particular note, risks were just as great in women using combined estrogen/progestin regimens as in women using estrogen alone, indicating that the regimens routinely prescribed to protect the uterus offer no protection against breast cancer.

More reassuring, and in direct contrast to these findings, were the results of another study, published soon after. The authors compared histories of postmenopausal estrogen/progestin use among 537 women who had breast cancer with those of 492 healthy control subjects. Researchers found no increased risk of breast cancer among women who took hormones for more than eight years. However, the number of breast cancer cases in this study was much smaller than in the Nurses' Health Study, in which there were 1,935 cases, and there were fewer long-term estrogen users. Therefore, the authors could not completely rule out a link between increased breast-cancer risk and postmenopausal hormone use (especially if taken on a long-term basis). However, the research team argued strongly against the possibility that there were any major increases in risk. Authors of an editorial that accompanied this second report took into account both these and other studies, and they were reassuring regarding any increases in breast-cancer risk that might be associated with postmenopausal hormone use.

How to Decide

Once a woman is aware of the risks and benefits of postmenopausal estrogen replacement, she should consider how these risks affect her. Coronary artery disease affects one in seven women 65 and older and accounts for about 250,000 deaths in U.S. women annually. Breast cancer, meanwhile, affects one in nine women over a lifetime and accounts for 45,000 deaths of U.S. women per year. Thus, even if estrogen-replacement therapy increased the much smaller risk of breast cancer by 50%, the reduction in the risk of coronary artery disease (of 40-50%) would tip the overall balance in favor of estrogen replacement for many women. The strongest indications for estrogen-replacement therapy would be for women with risk factors for coronary artery disease—high cholesterol, diabetes, high blood pressure, or a family history of early heart disease in a first-degree relative (parent, sister, or brother).

On the other hand, estrogen-replacement therapy is probably a bad idea for women with a personal history of breast cancer and may also be inappropriate for women who have a family history of breast cancer. In these women, the risks of estrogen therapy might come close to equaling the benefits—or might even outweigh them.

Recommendations are least clear for women with no particular risk factors for either coronary artery disease or breast cancer. Statistically, such women are much more likely to develop coronary disease than breast cancer. Investigators who have performed "decision analyses" to weigh the risks and benefits have suggested an expected net benefit if these women take hormones, but this remains uncertain.

Recommendations

At this point, there is no absolute answer to whether an individual woman should use postmenopausal hormone replacement. Scientists are, however, continuing to pursue the question. Currently under way is the Women's Health Initiative, the largest study ever launched to examine major causes of disease and death in postmenopausal women. One part of this study is a randomized trial of hormone replacement, which will involve 27,500 women nationwide. Women with an intact uterus are being assigned to take either combined estrogen/progestin therapy (Premarin 6.25 mg and Provera 2.5 mg daily) or a placebo (an inert pill); women who have had a hysterectomy (for whom there is no known benefit to adding a progestin) will take estrogen or a placebo. Treatment will continue for nine years, unless clear answers emerge sooner when experts meet periodically to review interim data. With close monitoring of the women for new cases of coronary artery disease, breast cancer, and fractures—in both the active-treatment and placebo groups—investigators expect to find out the true benefits and risks of hormone-replacement therapy for different groups of women.

What should women do while awaiting the results of the Women's Health Initiative? Many women will want to make a decision soon— especially the one-third of the female population who have already passed menopause. For now, each woman and her health-care provider should use the large body of information available to decide on the most rational approach for her.

Chapter 27

Postmenopausal Hormones— More Pros and Cons

A new study shows that women who take hormones live longer, and this benefit had the greatest impact on those at high risk for developing heart disease (*The New England Journal of Medicine*, 19 June 1997). A 37% lower death rate was shown among those who took hormones compared with those who did not. This good news, however, was offset by the finding that this protective effect diminished five years after the women stopped taking hormones. And current users received no additional benefit by continuing beyond the ten-year point. Worse, there was a 43% increase in breast cancer deaths among women who took hormones ten years or longer.

The study, conducted by Francine Grodstein, Sc.D., and colleagues at several Harvard-affiliated Medical Centers, is the first to look at overall survival rather than separating out the survival rates from heart disease, breast cancer, or hip fracture. The results call into question the standard medical advice to women that hormone therapy should begin at menopause and continue indefinitely. For mid-life women, the dilemma seems to boil down to this: Would I rather die of heart disease, hip fracture complications, or cancer? As noted in earlier issues of *HealthFacts,* estrogen reduces your odds of developing heart disease or fracture, but a certain proportion of women will develop these conditions despite long-term estrogen use.

The new findings, which also throw more heat than light on the question of how long to take hormones, come from the Nurses Health

HealthFacts, July 1997, Vol. 22, No.7, Pg. 1(2), © 1997 Center for Medical Consumers Inc.; reprinted with permission.

Study. Nearly 122,000 nurses, who were between the ages of 30 and 55 years when the study began in 1976, have answered extensive questionnaires every two years about their health, drug use, diet and other lifestyle factors. The majority of the hormone users took estrogen alone and a small group took the combination of estrogen and progestin. (The latter hormone is added to protect the uterus from estrogen-induced endometrial cancer.)

While the Nurses Health Study provides a gold mine of data regarding the health of older women, it does not provide definitive answers about hormone use. "There continues to be lingering questions regarding the extent to which reductions in mortality are due to hormone use itself as opposed to the characteristics of the user," wrote Drs. Louise A. Brinton and Catherine Schairer of the National Cancer Institute, in an editorial that accompanied the new study. They are referring to the well-documented observation that women who take hormones tend to be in an upper income bracket which, in itself, is associated with lower rates of heart disease, better health, and increased longevity.

Definitive answers to questions about the long-term safety and efficacy of hormones are not expected for at least ten more years. They will come from the ongoing government-sponsored clinical trial in which women have been randomly assigned to take either a placebo, estrogen, or estrogen plus progestin.

For the women who must make decisions now, Drs. Brinton and Schairer suggest that hormone therapy be considered by those at high risk for heart disease. They acknowledge, however, that hormones beneficial effects are dependent on recent use, and this raises questions about when to start the drug. Most gynecologists recommend starting at menopause. But a study published earlier this year contradicted this advice as it applies to the prevention of bone loss (see *HealthFacts*, March 1997). Estrogen's ability to preserve bone density lasts only as long as women take the drug. Those who did not start taking hormones until they were in their late sixties had about the same level of bone density by their seventies as those who started at menopause and never stopped.

Starting hormones later in life may also be the way to go for women at high risk for heart disease. Whether they decide to take hormones or not, older women should stop smoking, increase their physical activity, lower their fat intake, and so forth, because there are many ways to cut the risk of heart disease without resorting to drugs.

Unfortunately, the same cannot be said about breast cancer. Those at high risk for breast cancer would want to think twice about taking hormones longer than a few years for most studies show that the increased incidence of this disease begins after five years of estrogen use.

To recap the limited evidence on estrogen use: It may decrease the risk of heart disease, bone-thinning, fracture, and Alzheimer's disease. It is implicated in the development of endometrial cancer, breast cancer, gall bladder disease, asthma, lupus, mood disorders, facial pain, enlarged uterine fibroid tumors, vein clots, migraines, and kidney disease.

Lost in the debate over whether women should take hormones is a study that was published several months ago in the *Journal of the American Medical Association* (24 April 1997). Lawrence H. Kushi, Sc.D. and colleagues at the University of Minnesota School of Public Health, studied over 40,000 women, aged 55 to 69, for seven years. They found that regular exercise reduced the women's risk of premature death by 30%. This is close to the reduction in heart disease deaths achieved by estrogen without the increased risk of estrogen-induced breast cancer.

Chapter 28

Halt Heart Disease or Beat Breast Cancer: A Woman's Quandary

One is perceived to be the biggest health threat to women; the other is the real thing. Though both claim far too many lives, the 46,000 American women who die each year from breast cancer are but a small percentage of the 370,000 who succumb to this country's number one killer—heart disease. The truth is, after age 50, heart disease doesn't discriminate by gender.

Heart disease affects more than nine million American women in all, so it makes sense to seek protection. But sometimes reports in the media can be confusing for those trying to eat right to keep both heart disease and breast cancer at bay.

Already this year, researchers have released the results of two separate but equally compelling studies on diet and breast cancer that seem to sneer at current heart-healthy recommendations. What's a woman to do? First, don't panic. There's much more dietary advice in common for preventing the two diseases than you might think. But first, let's look at the two major areas of contention—fat and alcohol.

Fickle Finger of Fat

For decades, researchers have been playing tug-of-war with the implications of fat intake on breast cancer risk. It made sense at first

Environmental Nutrition, May 1998, Vol. 21, No.5, Pg. 1(2); © 1998 Environmental Nutrition Inc., 52 Riverside Drive, Suite 15A, New York, NY 10024; reprinted with permission.

to indict dietary fat. After all, countries with the highest rates of breast cancer also have the highest intakes of fat.

But the fat-breast cancer link was knocked down a peg in 1992 by Harvard researchers. After studying 80,000 women for eight years, they found no difference in risk between those who ate half their calories as fat and those who ate 30% as fat. Still, critics argue that a truly low-fat diet—under 25%—would be protective.

Now, a study from Sweden also suggests that a high-fat intake does not contribute to breast cancer. The study followed more than 61,000 Swedish women age 40 to 76 for more than four years. There was no correlation between the amount of fat the women consumed and their risk of breast cancer.

This time, however, the researchers went a step further and analyzed the results by the type of fat. Bingo! A more telling pattern emerged. Risk of breast cancer was lower in women who ate a diet high in monounsaturated fats—found in olive oil, canola oil and nuts. For every 10 grams of monounsaturated fat they ate, their risk fell by 45%.

Conversely, polyunsaturated fats were linked to increased risk. For each five grams eaten, risk rose by almost 70%. Poly fats include omega-6 fats like those found in vegetable oils as well as omega-3 fats found in fish oil. Though the study did not differentiate among individual fatty acids, a recent study found omega-3 fats protective against breast cancer, so presumably the omega-6 fats are the guilty ones.

The upshot for breast cancer seems to be that total fat intake doesn't really matter, though poly fats might be worse than other fats and mono fats might be better. At one time, this might have seemed to be heart-healthy advice turned upside-down. In fact, heart-healthy advice itself has been turned on its head of late.

Heart Disease Do's and Don'ts

Until now, heart-healthy advice has been mostly ad nauseum admonitions to cut back total fat calories to 30%. More recently, the message to reduce saturated fat has picked up steam as the dietary component considered to be most responsible for raising blood cholesterol levels, and thereby risk of heart disease. And lately, bans fatty acids have garnered suspicion as an additional anathema.

But as with breast cancer, new evidence is mounting that total fat intake may not be so important to heart disease risk, if the fat eaten is mostly mono (with little saturated or bans fats) and if calories are not excessive. For now though, most experts still recommend keeping fat under 30% of calories.

Alcohol: The Red Herring?

You'd think red wine was on the food pyramid these days, with all the glowing reports it's been getting. Experts think red wine protects against heart disease by supplying antioxidant compounds. Called phenols, they reduce the stickiness of blood, preventing dangerous coagulation. Whether alcohol itself has additional positive effects is still debated. There's been so much positive news about red wine that some doctors actually prescribe it. But not to women.

Until now, studies have merely suggested that alcohol increases breast cancer risk. But a new analysis that pooled the results from six studies involving more than 300,000 women has confirmed a strong link between alcohol and breast cancer. Risk of breast cancer increased 9% for those consuming 3/4 to one drink a day. Women who drank two to five drinks a day had a 41% increased risk compared to nondrinkers. Stephanie Smith-Warner, Ph.D., the study's lead researcher explains, "This risk is similar to the risk of women with a family history of breast cancer."

But before you swear off your nightcap, consider this: The American Cancer Society analyzed more than 500,000 middle-aged and older Americans for the link between alcohol and health. Those who consumed one drink a day had a 30% to 40% lower death rate from cardiovascular diseases and a 20% lower overall death rate.

Because so many more women die of heart disease than breast cancer, the odds favor erring on the side of preventing heart disease. If you do, limit alcohol to no more than one drink a day—that is, unless you already are at risk for breast cancer, because of family history, for instance.

Perhaps grape juice is the best of both worlds. It contains the beneficial phenols but no alcohol. A small study from the University of Wisconsin Medical Center recently found reduced clotting in those who consumed grape juice, similar to what's seen with red wine.

Common Sense Revisited: Bottom line?

The good news is that, for the most part, there's no need to sacrifice the risk of one disease for the other. Most nutrition advice for heart disease and breast cancer does not conflict. In only one area is advice truly conflicting—alcohol. EN suggests you weigh your personal risk factors before making a decision.

Don't forget, however, to also eat plenty of fruits and vegetables, maintain a desirable body weight and increase fiber intake. All are

Table 28.1 Heart vs. Breast: Weighing Healthful Choices

Diet Component	Heart Smart
Total Fat	Decrease total intake to 30% of calories or less or concentrate on improving mix of fats (more mono, less saturated and trans).
Omega-6 fats	Neutral effect.
Omega-3 fats	Beneficial. Increase consumption of fish, walnuts and flaxseed.
Monounsaturated fats	Beneficial. Increase consumption of olive oil, canola oil and peanuts.
Saturated fats	Reduce consumption of meats, butter and full-fat dairy.
Trans fats	Reduce consumption of stick margarine and processed snacks.
Fiber	Increase intake of soluble fiber (fruits, vegetables, legumes).
Alcohol	Moderate consumption (1-2 drinks a day) may be beneficial.
Weight	Reduce weight to decrease risk.
Folic acid	Get 400 micrograms from food (legumes, leafy greens, orange juice) and a multivitamin.

still good moves to help prevent both diseases. Check out our chart below to put it all together.

— by Catherine Golub

Table 28.1 Heart vs. Breast: Weighing Healthful Choices (continued)

Diet Component	Best for Breast
Total Fat	Overall intake may not be important but it may be best to keep intake moderate (30%) until more is known.
Omega-6 fats	May increase risk; limit vegetable oils and margarine.
Omega-3 fats	Preliminary research shows benefit; further research needed.
Monounsaturated fats	May be beneficial; further research needed.
Saturated fats	(Follow Heart-Smart advice.)
Trans fats	(Follow Heart-Smart advice.)
Fiber	Increase intake of both soluble and insoluble (bran) fiber.
Alcohol	Limit to 1 drink a day or abstain if at high risk for breast cancer.
Weight	Maintain desirable weight throughout adulthood to decrease risk.
Folic acid	(Follow Heart-Smart advice.)

Chapter 29

Synthetic Estrogens: Questions and Answers

What Is Premarin?

Premarin is the brand name of conjugated estrogens, manufactured by Wyeth-Ayerst, and derived from the urine of pregnant mares.

Who Takes Premarin and Why?

More than 8 million American women take Premarin each year for estrogen replacement to treat symptoms of menopause or to prevent and treat osteoporosis.

Is Premarin Somehow Better Than Other Estrogen Products? If Not, Why Is it So Widely Prescribed?

Premarin is different from other estrogen products in that it is the only brand of conjugated estrogens marketed in the U.S.[1] Other drugs approved for hormone replacement therapy contain different types of synthetic estrogens, including dienestrol, estradiol, esterified estrogens, and estropipate.

Despite the different composition of these drugs, they have all been demonstrated to be safe and effective for the treatment of menopausal symptoms and many of them have been found to be safe and effective

---

"Synthetic Conjugated Estrogens: Questions and Answers," from http:// www.fda.gov/cder/news/ceqa.htm, May 1997, United States Food and Drug Administration (FDA), Center for Drug Evaluation and Research.

for prevention of osteoporosis too. Premarin has not been demonstrated to be superior to other marketed products.

Various factors affect the prescribing habits and preferences of physicians. Among these are manufacturer's advertising and promotional techniques as well as patient's knowledge and request for commonly used products.

What Is a Generic Drug?

A generic drug is a "copy" of a brand-name drug. The Federal Food, Drug, and Cosmetic Act (FD&C Act) states that the application for marketing a generic drug, called an Abbreviated New Drug Application or ANDA, must contain, among other things, information to show that the active ingredient of the new drug is the same as that of the listed drug. The Act goes on to say that the generic copy should be approved for marketing unless "the information submitted with the application is insufficient to show that the active ingredients are the same as the active ingredients of the listed drug."

How Is a Generic Drug Evaluated and Approved?

The FD&C Act requires that a generic copy contain, among other things, the same active ingredients as the reference listed drug (usually the innovator or brand name drug.) Additionally, the generic copy must be demonstrated to be bioequivalent to—that is, shown to be absorbed and used by the body in the same way as—the reference listed drug.

New, or innovator, drugs require an evaluation of safety and effectiveness in human trials. Generic drug manufacturers are not required to replicate this extensive clinical testing. Instead, a generic drug must be shown to be the same as the innovator drug and, therefore, can be expected to have the same effects as the innovator drug.

The Center for Drug Evaluation and Research (CDER) reviews generic drug marketing applications. Scientific staff in CDER review all applications for their scientific content, manufacturing procedures, and labeling claims.

What Is CDER's Position on Generic Premarin?

CDER concludes that an abbreviated new drug application (ANDA) for a synthetic version of Premarin cannot be approved at this time because the active ingredients in Premarin have not yet been adequately defined.

Doesn't a Generic Product Just Have to Conform to the Current USP Drug Substance Monograph?

To be approved for marketing, a generic product must have the same active ingredients as the reference listed drug. Compliance with the USP monograph is not a legal requirement for the approval of an ANDA, nor is compliance with the monograph necessarily sufficient to determine whether the statutory requirements of the FD&C Act for the approval of a generic drug have been fulfilled. FDA applies current scientific knowledge in making its approval decisions, even if that knowledge has not yet been incorporated into the USP monograph.

FDA Had Consistently Supported the Position Taken in the 1970 USP Monograph That the Ingredients Sodium Estrone Sulfate and Sodium Equilin Sulfate Are the Sole Active Ingredients in Premarin. Doesn't This Reverse That Position?

Yes. At the time of publication of the monograph in 1970, little information was available on the effects of estrogens on bone and the estimates of estrogenic potency of Premarin components were derived from clinical studies of menopausal symptoms. In addition, data on the detailed composition of Premarin and the pharmacologic activity of its components were limited. In fact, at the time, much of the available data indicated that many compounds found in Premarin were present in small amounts, and had weak estrogenic activity—characteristics associated with impurities. Premarin was, therefore, defined in terms of the total estrogenic potency of the two active ingredients rather than the sum of the potencies of various components.

Since that time, emerging scientific evidence demonstrates that all estrogens do not exert their effects in a uniform manner with respect to different target tissues. Newer analytical techniques applied to determine the composition of Premarin now demonstrate that it consists of a mixture of a substantial number of compounds with potential pharmacologic activity.

Clinical studies performed since publication of the USP monograph reveal that the assigned potencies of the components of Premarin tablets do not correctly reflect their relative potencies, and that at least one ingredient, previously believed to be an impurity, actually generates a significant concentration of a potentially active metabolite.

Based on new scientific information as well as improved techniques for compositional analysis, CDER can no longer support the position taken in the current USP monograph.

What Data Have Been Submitted to Demonstrate That an Approved ANDA Meeting the USP Monograph for Synthetic Conjugated Estrogens Tablets Would Not Provide the Same Clinical Effects As Premarin?

The statute does not require that the generic drug have the same clinical effects, nor does it require clinical trials demonstrating the generic drugs safety and efficacy. The safety and effectiveness of the generic are assured by showing that, among other things, the generic drug has the same active ingredients as the innovator. Because evidence presented to the agency demonstrates Premarin may have active ingredients in addition to those identified in the USP monograph, the agency cannot at this time approve an ANDA for a synthetic form of conjugated estrogens unless the active ingredients in Premarin are adequately identified and the ANDA demonstrates that the generic product contains the same ingredients.

What Will Happen to the USP Monograph for Conjugated Estrogens?

CDER is considering making recommendations to the USP regarding the current scientific information about the composition of conjugated estrogens.

Why Was This Position Not Discussed with an Advisory Committee?

The issue of the active ingredients in Premarin was discussed in 1989 with FDA's Fertility and Maternal Health Drugs Advisory Committee, in 1990 with an ad hoc subcommittee of this same committee, and in 1995 with this committee plus representation from FDA's Generic Drugs Advisory Committee and FDA's Endocrinologic and Metabolic Drugs Advisory Committee. Following each of these meetings, the Committee was unable to determine whether or not any individual component of Premarin or any combination of components other than estrone sulfate and equilin sulfate must be present in order for Premarin to achieve its established levels of efficacy and safety.

CDER's position regarding the approvability of generic conjugated estrogens at this time is consistent with the findings of the Advisory Committee; the position is based upon the fact that the active ingredients in Premarin have not yet been defined.

Will a Generic of Premarin Ever Be Approved?

Approval of a generic copy of Premarin would result in significant cost savings for American women, an outcome strongly supported by the FDA. Approval of a generic copy of Premarin will require an assurance that such copies contain the same active ingredients as Premarin. It is both feasible and desirable for the constituent active ingredients of Premarin to be characterized to this extent and Wyeth-Ayerst has committed to so characterize the active ingredients in Premarin.

Why Has This Announcement Taken So Long?

Over the years, there has been considerable controversy about the required composition and testing of generic conjugated estrogens. The decision to approve a generic version of any drug, especially one in such widespread use, has profound medical and regulatory implications. The determination of bioequivalence upon which a generic approval is based must be supported by strong science. Newly available information about the composition of Premarin from modern analytical techniques coupled with the results from new clinical studies had to be thoroughly evaluated to be certain that a decision on whether or not to approve applications for generic Premarin was firmly grounded in sound, up-to-date science.

Fact-finding in the face of emerging new information adds significant time to the process. All available information has to be thoroughly considered to be as certain as current science allows that positions taken are in the best interest of the public health.

Is There Consensus Within the FDA for This Position?

Although support for CDER's approach has not been unanimous, the full range of views and evidence was thoroughly considered in reaching CDER's position.

Has There Been External Pressure (from Wyeth-Ayerst, Congress, the Generic Manufacturers) to Influence This Position?

Issues with this level of public interest often stimulate interested parties to provide information to influence CDER. CDER considers all relevant information, regardless of its source, when considering important matters.

Could FDA Approve Generic Copies of Premarin Made from the Pregnant Mares' Urine?

Despite the fact that Premarin is not adequately characterized at this time, the Agency could approve generic copies of Premarin that originate from the same source material (pregnant mares' urine). This is because the reference listed drug is manufactured and controlled using these methods, and there could be confidence that generic copies using the same source materials and controlled in the same manner would have the same level of assurance that the same active ingredients are in the generic product as are in Premarin.

Isn't the FDA Concerned about the Cruelty Inflicted upon Pregnant Mares in the Making of Premarin?

A number of approved synthetic drug products, including piperazine estrone sulfate, micronized estradiol, and transdermal estradiol patches, are approved for the same indications as Premarin and are not derived from animal sources.

In addition, FDA encourages the initiation of studies that will permit the scientific determination of the active ingredients in Premarin and allow potential approval of synthetic generic versions of the drug. Once Premarin has been sufficiently characterized, FDA is committed to the expeditious review and approval of synthetic generic conjugated estrogens with the same active ingredients as, bioequivalent to, and thus assured to be as safe and effective as, Premarin.

Does FDA Intend to Answer Wyeth-Ayerst's Citizen Petition, or Does Today's Announcement Effectively Answer the Petition?

Today's announcement provides CDER's current position on the approvability of applications for generic synthetic conjugated estrogens drug products. Along with the announcement, CDER has made public a detailed memorandum regarding the approvability of a generic version of Premarin. CDER expects to receive comments on the announcement and underlying memorandum. If comments on the announcement and underlying memorandum are submitted to the Wyeth-Ayerst citizen petition docket, the agency will consider those comments in responding to the petition. The timing of FDA's petition response will depend, in part, on the volume of new comments and submissions received after the release of the announcement and memorandum.

Editorial Note

1. In 1999, the FDA also approved Cenestin™, a plant-derived conjugated estrogen product, produced by Duramed Pharmaceuticals.

Part Five

Dietary Issues and Cardiac Health

Chapter 30

Women and Nutrition: A Menu of Special Needs

Breast cancer. Osteoporosis. Iron deficiency. Weight reduction. What do these things have in common? They are either unique to women, or are more prevalent in women. And they affect current recommendations on what women should eat for optimum health.

While new information on what's good and what's bad seems to surface almost daily, some basic guidelines have taken root over the past several years.

The bottom line (also known as the Dietary Guidelines for Americans, from the Departments of Health and Human Services and Agriculture) is:

- eat a variety of foods
- maintain healthy weight
- choose a diet low in fat, saturated fat, and cholesterol
- choose a diet with plenty of vegetables, fruits, and grain products
- use sugar and salt/sodium only in moderation
- if you drink alcoholic beverages, do so in moderation.

That sounds simple enough. Except, what exactly is variety? Cake one day, cookies the next? What is a diet low in fat, saturated fat, and cholesterol? And, finally, what parts of a healthy diet have special importance for women?

FDA Consumer, January-February 1991, Publication No. (FDA) 91-2247, reprinted in May 1995.

Vitamins and Minerals

There are several vitamins and minerals essential to a healthy diet. A well-balanced diet will usually meet women's allowances for them. (See Table 30.1) However, for good health, women need to pay special attention to two minerals, calcium and iron.

Calcium

Both women and men need enough calcium to build peak (maximum) bone mass during their early years of life. Low calcium intake appears to be one important factor in the development of osteoporosis. Women have a greater risk than men of developing osteoporosis.

A condition in which progressive loss of bone mass occurs with aging, osteoporosis causes the bones to be more susceptible to fracture. If a woman has a high level of bone mass when her skeleton matures, this may modify her risk of developing osteoporosis.

Therefore, particularly during adolescence and early adulthood, women should increase their food sources of calcium. "The most important time to get a sufficient amount of calcium is while bone growth and consolidation are occurring, a period that continues until approximately age 30 to 35," says Marilyn Stephenson, a registered dietitian with FDA's Center for Food Safety and Applied Nutrition. "The idea is, if you can build a maximum peak of calcium deposits early on, this may delay fractures that occur later in life."

The recommended dietary allowance (RDA) for calcium for woman 19 to 24 is 1,200 milligrams per day. For women 25 and older, the allowance drops to 800 milligrams, but that is still a significant amount, says Stephenson. "The need for good dietary sources of calcium continues throughout life," she says.

How do you get enough calcium without too many calories and fat? After all, the foods that top the calcium charts—milk, cheese, ice cream—aren't calorie and fat lightweights.

"There are lots of lower fat choices," says Stephenson. "There's 1 percent or skim milk instead of whole milk. There's a good variety of lower fat cheeses, yogurts, and frozen yogurts, and there's a whole flock of substitutes for ice cream."

In addition to dairy foods, other good sources of calcium include salmon, tofu (soybean curd), certain vegetables (for example, broccoli), legumes (peas and beans), calcium-enriched grain products, lime-processed tortillas, seeds, and nuts.

228

Iron

For women, the RDA for iron is 15 milligrams per day, 5 milligrams more than the RDA for men. Women need more of this mineral because they lose an average of 15 to 20 milligrams of iron each month during menstruation. Without enough iron, iron deficiency anemia can develop and cause symptoms that include pallor, fatigue and headaches.

After menopause, body iron stores generally begin to increase. Therefore, iron deficiency in women over 50 may indicate blood loss from another source, and should be checked by a physician.

Animal products—meat, fish and poultry—are good and important sources of iron. In addition, the type of iron, known as heme iron, in these foods is well absorbed in the human intestine.

Dietary iron from plant sources, called non-heme, are found in peas and beans, spinach and other green leafy vegetables, potatoes, and whole-grain and iron-fortified cereal products. Although non-heme iron is not as well absorbed as heme iron, the amount of non-heme iron absorbed from a meal is influenced by other constituents in the diet. The addition of even relatively small amounts of meat or foods containing vitamin C substantially increases the total amount of iron absorbed from the entire meal.

Calories and Weight Control

The Food and Nutrition Board of the National Research Council recommends that the average woman between 23 and 50 eat about 2,200 calories a day to maintain weight. (See Table 30.2)

The best way for a woman to determine whether she's eating the right number of calories is to "keep stepping on the scale," says FDA's Stephenson. She cautions, however, that cutting back on calories isn't always the answer to losing weight. "You don't really want to cut back any more [calories] if you're down around that [1,500 calories] range," says Stephenson. She explains that the fewer the calories you have to work with, the harder it is to meet all your daily requirements for a healthy diet.

"If you find you are gaining weight, you need to think of not only cutting calories, but also about increasing exercise," she says. "Calories are only half the equation for weight control. Physical activity burns calories, increases the proportion of lean to fat body mass, and raises your metabolism. So, a combination of both calorie control and increased physical activity is important for attaining healthy weight.

229

On the other hand, if you've been pigging out—well, you know what you have to do."

Cholesterol

Women tend to have higher levels than men of a desirable type of cholesterol called HDLs (high-density lipoproteins) until menopause, leading some researchers to believe there is a link between HDLs and estrogen levels. But this doesn't let women off the hook—a diet high in saturated fat and cholesterol can still mean trouble.

For both women and men, blood cholesterol levels of below 200 milligrams are desirable. Levels between 200 and 239 milligrams are considered borderline, and anything over 240 milligrams is high. High levels of blood cholesterol increase the risk of coronary heart disease. To keep levels in the good range, the National Cholesterol Education Program of the National Heart, Lung, and Blood Institute recommends eating no more than 300 milligrams of cholesterol a day. Cholesterol is found only in food from animal sources, such as egg yolks, dairy products, meat, poultry, shellfish, and—in smaller amounts—fish and some processed products containing animal foods.

Even more important than limiting cholesterol to under 300 milligrams is keeping saturated fat to under 10 percent of total calories, says Nancy Ernst, the nutrition coordinator for the National Heart, Lung, and Blood Institute. "Don't even think about cholesterol in your diet," says Ernst. "Focus on reducing saturated fat."

Fat

In the United States, out of every 100,000 women, approximately 27 die from breast cancer each year. In Japan, breast cancer deaths are fewer than 7 per 100,000. Some scientists think that the difference in death rates may be related to the different amounts of fat in the average diet in each country—40 percent for American women versus 20 percent in Japan.

"We believe pretty strongly in the link [between high-fat diets and breast cancer]," says Jeffrey McKenna, director of NCI's Cancer Awareness Program. Population studies have also linked high-fat diets to other cancers, particularly colorectal cancer.

Fat does, however, serve a purpose in the diet. Fats in foods provide energy and help the body absorb certain vitamins. But it is as easy as pie (and doughnuts, ice cream, and sirloin steaks) to eat too much.

For a healthy diet, the diet and health report of the National Research Council recommends reducing fat to no more than 30 percent of total calories. But that's not all. In terms of heart disease, the kinds of fat you eat are as important as how much.

There are three kinds of fat—saturated, polyunsaturated and monounsaturated. All three are equal when it comes to calories—9 per gram (compared to 4 calories per gram for protein or carbohydrate). But they aren't equal when it comes to how they affect your health.

More than anything else in the diet, saturated fat can raise your blood cholesterol level. Because of this risk, less than one-third of your daily fat intake (less than 10 percent of total calories) should come from saturated fats.

That's the bad news. The good news is polyunsaturated and monounsaturated may actually lower blood cholesterol levels. The diet and health report recommends that not more than 10 percent of total calories should be from polyunsaturated fat, and monounsaturated fat should make up the remaining 10 percent.

The foods with the highest amounts of saturated fat come from animals—meat, of course, and foods derived from animals, such as butter, cream, ice cream, and cheese. In addition to animal products, coconut and palm kernel oils are very high in saturated fat—over 90 percent. The best sources for polyunsaturated fats are plant-based oils—sunflower, corn, soybean, cottonseed, and safflower. Monounsaturated fats are found in the largest amounts in olive, canola and peanut oils.

Figure Out Your Fat Intake

The recommendation is that no more than 30 percent of total calories come from fat. Food labels list fat in grams. To find out what your total intake of fats in grams should be limited to, multiply your daily calories by 0.30 (30 percent) and divide by 9 (the number of calories in a gram of fat).

Example:

2,200 calories times 0.30 = 660 calories from fat
660 calories divided by 9 = 73 grams of fat

Fiber

An apple a day—that is, a whole apple with the skin—will give you approximately 3.6 grams of fiber. That's a good start, but you still need

Table 30.1 National Academy of Sciences/National Research Council Recommended Dietary Allowances for Women Age 19 to 50 (1989)

Vitamins

Vitamin A:	800 micrograms
Vitamin D:	10 micrograms (age 19 to 24), 5 micrograms (age 25 to 50)
Vitamin E:	8 milligrams
Vitamin K:	60 micrograms (19 to 24), 65 micrograms (25 to 50)
Vitamin C:	60 milligrams
Thiamine:	1.1 milligrams
Riboflavin:	1.3 milligrams
Niacin:	15 milligrams
Vitamin B6:	1.6 milligrams
Folate:	180 micrograms
Vitamin B12:	2 micrograms

Minerals

Calcium:	1,200 milligrams (19 to 24), 800 milligrams (25 to 50)
Phosphorus:	1,200 milligrams (19 to 24), 800 milligrams (25 to 50)
Magnesium:	280 milligrams
Iron:	15 milligrams
Zinc:	12 milligrams
Iodine:	150 micrograms
Selenium:	55 micrograms

Table 30.2 Suggested Weights for Adults

Age 19 to 34		*Age 35 and over*	
Height	Weight (in pounds)	Height	Weight (in pounds)
5'0"	97-128	5'0"	108-138
5'1"	101-132	5'1"	111-143
5'2"	104-137	5'2"	115-148
5'3"	107-141	5'3"	119-152
5'4"	111-146	5'4"	122-157
5'5"	114-150	5'5"	126-162
5'6"	118-155	5'6"	130-167
5'7"	121-160	5'7"	134-172
5'8"	125-164	5'8"	138-178
5'9"	129-169	5'9"	142-183
5'10"	132-174	5'10"	146-188
5'11"	136-179	5'11"	151-194
6'0"	140-184	6'0"	155-199
6'1"	144-189	6'1"	159-205
6'2"	148-195	6'2"	165-210
6'3"	152-200	6'3"	168-216
6'4"	156-205	6'4"	173-222
6'5"	160-211	6'5"	177-228
6'6"	164-216	6'6"	182-234

Height without shoes

Weight without clothes

The higher weights in the ranges generally apply to men, who tend to have larger body frames and more muscle; the lower weights more often apply to women, who have smaller body frames and less muscle. Weights even below the range may be appropriate for some small-boned people.

(Source: National Research Council, 1989)

a lot more fruits, vegetables, and whole grains to meet the daily level of 20 to 30 grams of fiber recommended by the National Cancer Institute. Eating foods with plenty of complex carbohydrates and fiber (vegetables, fruits, and grain products) is part of a healthy diet for several reasons. A fiber-rich diet is helpful in the management of constipation and may be related to lower rates of colon cancer. These types of foods are generally low in fat and can be substitutes for fatty foods.

Fiber comes in two forms—insoluble and soluble. Insoluble fiber, mostly found in whole-grain products, vegetables and fruit, provides bulk for stool formation and helps move wastes more quickly through the colon. Another benefit is the full feeling fiber may create in the stomach, a possible deterrent to overeating.

Soluble fiber has been linked to lowering blood cholesterol levels, but that's still a research area according to the Surgeon General's Report on Nutrition and Health. There are many sources of soluble fiber, including peas and beans, many vegetables and fruits, and rice, corn and oat bran. There are even small amounts in pasta, crackers, and other bakery products.

Although foods containing fiber seem to exert a protective effect against some cancers, the diet and health report points out there is no conclusive evidence that dietary fiber itself, rather than other components, exerts this effect. Therefore, the report does not recommend the use of fiber supplements.

As important as fiber is to good health, it can be overdone. NCI recommends an upper limit of 35 grams a day. More probably won't further increase the benefits from fiber, and may interfere with the body's ability to absorb iron and other minerals.

When increasing the amount of fiber in your diet, do it slowly, so your body can become accustomed to handling it. Adding too much fiber too quickly may lead to uncomfortable side effects, including abdominal discomfort, flatulence and diarrhea.

Food Preparation

Carefully selecting foods for a well-balanced diet can end up a wasted effort if equal care isn't used in the kitchen. Some important points to help make the most of healthy food: To help reduce fat, broil, bake or microwave food rather than frying or deep-fat frying. Cook vegetables in as little water as possible, or, instead of boiling food, try steaming. The steamer basket keeps the food above the water so the nutrients can't be washed away. Also, heat can destroy some nutrients, so don't overcook. Use fresh foods as soon as possible to avoid loss of vitamins. Season vegetables with herbs and spices instead of high-fat sauces, butter or margarine. Try lemon juice as a salad dressing. Substitute plain low-fat yogurt, blender-whipped low-fat cottage cheese, or buttermilk in recipes that call for sour cream or mayonnaise. Use skim or low-fat milk in place of whole milk in puddings, soups, and baked products.

Getting a Variety of Foods

The Dietary Guidelines say that the many nutrients you need should come from a variety of foods, not from a few highly fortified foods or supplements. A good way to ensure variety is to choose foods each day from the five major food groups. USDA has developed a daily food guide for a well-balanced diet that suggests the following:

- vegetables—3 to 5 servings
- fruits—2 to 4 servings
- breads, cereals, rice, pasta—6 to 11 servings
- milk, yogurt, cheese—2 to 3 servings
- meat, poultry, fish, dried beans and peas, eggs, nuts—2 to 3 servings

This food guide is "a useful, simple way for women to look at their own diets and see how to improve them," says Stephenson. By choosing different foods from each group daily, the food guide can serve as the basis for the dietary guideline "eat a variety of foods," says Stephenson, and "that's a tenet of nutritional advice for all people."

Finally, the guidelines are meant for the average person, cautions Walter H. Glinsmann, M.D., FDA's associate director for clinical nutrition. "Almost nobody is average," he says. Lifestyle, genetics, and conditions such as pregnancy or disease can also affect a person's nutritional needs, he explains.

—by Dori Stehlin

Dori Stehlin is a staff writer for *FDA Consumer*.

Chapter 31

Dietary Fiber

Coronary artery disease is responsible for the deaths of 240,000 women each year in the United States. However, changing one's lifestyle habits can have powerful effects on the development and progression of heart disease.

Recent scientific interest and subsequent studies have focused attention on the role fiber plays in diet. Dietary fiber, well known for its role in lowering the risk of colon cancer and diverticulosis (inflammation of the colon lining), has also been shown to lower serum cholesterol levels.

Since the turn of the century, the consumption of dietary fiber has decreased while the incidence of heart disease and colon cancer has climbed. Dietary fiber is part of the structure of plants and is found in grains, legumes, fruits and vegetables. It is not present in meat or dairy products.

There are Two Types of Fiber: Soluble *and* Insoluble.

Soluble fiber dissolves in water and forms a gel-like substance in the colon. Recent studies have shown that the ingestion of soluble fiber reduces cholesterol levels. When an average of 6 grams of soluble fiber is consumed daily, the average decrease in LDL cholesterol ("bad" cholesterol) levels was 14 percent for people with elevated cholesterol levels and 10 percent for those who had normal levels. When combined

"Dietary Fiber: Another Way to Lower Your Risk of Heart Disease," Information provided by the Norton Hospital Women's Pavilion Heart Center, © Norton Hospital, undated; reprinted with permission.

with a diet low in saturated fats and moderate exercise, the overall decrease can be substantial.

Insoluble fiber, better known as "roughage," does not dissolve in water. It adds bulk and helps move things along in the colon, reducing the risk of colon cancer.

The recommended dietary fiber intake is 20 to 30 grams per day. This level is easy to achieve by following the food pyramid recommendations of five or more servings of fruits/vegetables per day and six or more servings of grains per day. A word of advice: gradually increase the amount of dietary fiber to give your body time to adjust.

Mexican Grain Salad—A High Fiber Recipe

1/4 cup barley, uncooked
1/4 cup lime juice
2 Tbsp water
1 Tbsp olive oil
1 tsp sugar
1/2 tsp salt
1/2 tsp garlic powder
1/4 tsp black pepper
1/4 tsp ground cumin
1/4 tsp red pepper
1—15 oz can black beans, rinsed and drained
Leaf lettuce
1 cup chopped tomato
1/4 cup shredded fat free cheddar cheese
1/4 cup sliced green onions

Cook barley according to package directions; drain and set aside. Combine lime juice and next eight ingredients in a jar. Cover and shake vigorously.

Pour 1/2 of dressing over barley and mix well. In a separate bowl, combine beans and rest of dressing. Cover each and refrigerate eight hours. Spoon barley mixture evenly onto lettuce-lined plates. Top evenly with beans, tomato, cheese and green onions.

Servings: Four
Calories: 340
Fat: 5 gm
Cholesterol: 10 mg
Fiber: 10.8 gm
Sodium: 260 mg

Chapter 32

Homocysteine and Heart Disease

Homocysteine (pronounced homo-SIS-teen) is an amino acid and is found normally in the body. Its metabolism is linked to that of several vitamins, especially folic acid, B6, and B12. Deficiencies of those vitamins may cause elevated levels of homocysteine.

In recent years, studies have accumulated suggesting that a high level of homocysteine increases a person's chance of developing heart disease, stroke, and peripheral vascular disease (a reduced blood flow to the hands and feet).

In September 1995, the National Heart, Lung, and Blood Institute (NHLBI) convened a special panel to review the scientific evidence about homocysteine's possible link to heart disease. The information that follows is based on the panel's conclusions.

Briefly, the panel said that an elevated homocysteine level appears to increase the risk of heart disease, stroke, and peripheral vascular disease. However, no studies have been done to show that lowering the homocysteine level reduces the risk of heart disease. The panel stressed that more research, especially a clinical trial, must be done to understand the possible association between the level of homocysteine and heart and related diseases.

Homocysteine and Heart Disease

Various studies have found that persons with elevated levels of homocysteine in their blood are at an increased risk of heart and vessel

www.nhlbi.nih.gov/health/public/heart/other/homocyst.txt, March 13, 1996, from the National Heart, Lung, and Blood Institute (NHLBI).

disease. These studies include the Physicians' Health Study, the Tromso Study from Norway, the Framingham Heart Study, and a meta-analysis of nearly 40 studies.

Some studies indicate that persons with elevated homocysteine levels tend to also have other risk factors for heart disease, especially smoking, high blood pressure, and high blood cholesterol.

So far, no clinical trial has been done to show that lowering homocysteine levels alters the progression of heart disease, or prevents heart attacks or strokes.

Why Homocysteine?

Much more basic research must be done before scientists understand how an elevated homocysteine level affects the development and progression of heart disease. However, scientists have several theories: First, a high level of homocysteine may be involved with the process called atherosclerosis, the gradual buildup of fatty substances in arteries. Homocysteine also may make blood more likely to clot by increasing the stickiness of blood platelets. Clots can block blood flow, causing a heart attack or stroke. Increased homocysteine may affect other substances involved in clotting too. Finally, higher homocysteine levels may make blood vessels less flexible—and so less able to widen to increase blood flow. However, none of theories has so far been proven.

What Determines Homocysteine Levels?

Individuals differ in their levels of homocysteine. Two key factors affect a person's homocysteine level—genetics and environment.

Genetics

Genetic factors help regulate the level of homocysteine in the blood. For instance, genetic flaws (mutations) can affect homocysteine's metabolism. The NHLBI Family Heart Study found families with genetic mutations in the enzymes involved in homocysteine metabolism.

The NHLBI Framingham Heart Study and other investigations have found a relationship between elevated homocysteine levels and families with early heart disease.

Environment

The level of homocysteine in the blood also is affected by the consumption of vitamins, especially folic acid, B6, and B12.

Data from the Framingham Heart Study show that only 30-40 percent of the population was getting 200 or more micrograms of folic acid in their diet. The data indicated that for many persons an intake of at least 400 micrograms was needed to keep homocysteine levels from becoming elevated.

Data also indicate that homocysteine levels are higher in older persons than younger ones, and in women after menopause than in those before. But more research is needed to confirm and explain these differences.

Sources of Folic Acid, B6, and B12

Americans who follow a well-balanced diet should get enough vitamins, including folic acid, B6, and B12. There are no data to support the benefit of taking a folic acid supplement for heart and vessel diseases.

Some food sources of folic acid, B6, and B12 are given below. The list includes sample percentages of the recommended daily value (RDV) for each vitamin. These RDVs are: 400 micrograms for folic acid, 2 milligrams for B6, and 6 micrograms for B12.

Folic Acid, Also Called Folate

More than a third of the folic acid in most Americans' diet comes from citrus fruits, tomatoes, and vegetables. Grain products also are an important source of folic acid.

For example, 1/2-cup of spinach gives at least a third of the RDV for folic acid. A 1/2-cup of asparagus, broccoli, or green peas gives 10-24 percent of the RDV. An 8-ounce glass of orange juice and 1/2 cup of asparagus each has about a quarter of RDV.

Americans also can use beans and lentils as sources of folic acid. A 1/2-cup of black-eyed peas, lentils, lima beans, pinto beans, or navy beans gives at least a third of the RDV for folic acid.

Vitamin B6

Americans' major sources of vitamin B6 are meat, poultry, fish, fruits, vegetables, and grain products.

For example, 1 banana has up to 40 percent of the RDV for B6. One baked potato, a 1 3/4-cup serving of watermelon, or a 3-ounce serving of salmon or turkey gives up to a quarter of the RDV for B6.

Vitamin B12

Americans' major sources of vitamin B12 are meat, poultry, fish, and milk and milk products. B12 is not found in fruits, vegetables, beans, grains, nuts, or seeds.

For example, a 3-ounce serving of mackerel or trout has more than 40 percent of the RDV for B12. A 3-ounce serving of tuna has up to 40 percent of the RDV for B12. One cup of nonfat plain yogurt has about a quarter of the RDV for B12.

Some foods, such as breakfast cereals, have folic acid and other nutrients added to them. Check the food label for the RDV for folic acid.

Beginning in January 1998, certain foods [were] required by the U.S. Food and Drug Administration to add folic acid in order to help prevent birth defects, such as spina bifida. These foods include enriched breads and rolls, all enriched flours, corn meals, all enriched macaroni and noodle products, and breakfast cereals. Food labels may say the product has been fortified with folic acid.

What Lies Ahead?

It is not yet definitely known if elevated homocysteine is a risk factor for heart disease—that is, if it really increases a person's chance of developing heart disease. Known risk factors for heart disease are age (being 45 or older for men; 55 or older for women), a family history of early heart disease, high blood pressure, high blood cholesterol, smoking, obesity, physical inactivity, and diabetes.

Until more research is done, Americans can protect their health by following a heart-healthy food plan. Those concerned about homocysteine should talk to their doctor.

The September NHLBI panel called for more research to help answer the many questions about homocysteine's possible role in the development and progression of heart disease and stroke. These questions include:

- Does homocysteine damage blood vessel walls?

- What regulates the level of homocysteine in the blood and how?

- What happens to heart disease when homocysteine levels drop?

- What are the differences in homocysteine levels among men and pre- and post-menopausal women?

- If significant differences exist, why?

242

- Can keeping homocysteine levels low prevent heart disease and stroke?

- Can reducing homocysteine levels prevent repeat heart attacks?

- What is the best amount and of which vitamins to prevent heart attack and stroke?

- Does the homocysteine level interact with known modifiable risk factors for heart disease?

For More Information

A healthy eating plan supplies enough folic acid, B6, and B12. For more information about healthy eating, write to the NHLBI Information Center, P.O. Box 30105, Bethesda, MD 20824-0105.

Another source of information about healthy eating is: *"Nutrition and Your Health: Dietary Guidelines for Americans."* To get a copy, send $0.50 by check or money order made payable to the "Superintendent of Documents" to the Consumer Information Center, Department 378-C, Pueblo, CO 81009. The guidelines also are available for free from the Department of Health and Human Services Home Page on the World Wide Web at: http://www.os.dhhs.gov.

Chapter 33

Coffee and Coronary Disease in Women

Despite extensive investigation, the relationship between coffee intake and the risk of coronary heart disease remains controversial. Most case-control studies have shown a positive association, with a typical relative risk of 1.42 for consumption of five cups per day. Prospective studies, which are less prone to bias, have shown a weaker association, with a summary relative risk of only 1.18. This report describes the relationship between coffee intake and coronary risk in one of the largest ongoing prospective studies in women—the US Nurses' Health Study.

In this study, 85,747 women (aged 34-59 years) with no history of heart disease, stroke, or cancer provided information on coffee intake and other dietary factors in 1980. Coffee consumption varied greatly in the study population; 22% of the subjects consumed less than one cup of caffeinated coffee a month, while 17% consumed four to five cups a day and 8% consumed six or more cups a day.

During 10 years of follow-up, 712 cases of coronary heart disease occurred in the cohort. After adjustment for age, smoking and other risk factors, no association was found between coffee consumption and risk of coronary disease. Special analyses for the effects of recent coffee consumption, coffee consumption before 1976 (when percolation was the most common method of preparation), decaffeinated coffee

"Coffee and Coronary Disease in Women," in *Nutrition Research Newsletter*, March 1996, Vol. 15, No. 3, Pg. 30(1), © 1996 Lyda Associates Inc.; reprinted with permission.

intake, or total caffeine intake also showed no significant effects. Coffee consumption was strongly correlated with cigarette smoking.

These findings do not support the hypothesis that coffee drinking increases the risk of coronary disease in US women. The study had several important strengths which support the validity of its findings: the number of subjects was large, the study design was prospective, the subjects' coffee intakes varied widely, the follow-up rate was high, and extensive information was available about possible confounding factors. The authors point out that because coffee drinking is strongly associated with cigarette smoking, it is necessary to control carefully for this important cause of coronary disease. It is possible that the associations between coffee drinking and coronary disease seen in some previous studies may have reflected inadequate control for smoking rather than true effects of coffee itself.

Walter C. Willett, Meir J. Stampfer, Joann E. Manson et al, "Coffee Consumption and Coronary Heart Disease in Women. A Ten-Year Follow-up," *JAMA* 275(6): 458-462 (14 Feb 1996) [Reprints: Walter C Willett, MD, DRPH, Channing Laboratory, 818 Longwood Avenue, Boston MA 02115]

Additional Reading

J.J. Barone and H.R. Roberts, Caffeine Consumption [Review], *Food & Chemical Toxicology*, Pg.34(10):119-129 (Jan 1996) [Correspondence: J.J. Barone, The Coca-Cola Company, One Coca-Cola Plaza, Atlanta GA 30313]

Chapter 34

Shopping for a Healthy Heart

The battle against fat begins and ends in those well-stocked aisles of your local supermarket. The average grocery store is stocked with more than 20,000 food items. Based on these numbers, it is not surprising that most people are choosing the typical American diet—high in total fat, especially saturated fat, cholesterol, salt and calories. Being prepared to make healthier food choices at the supermarket, will automatically make it easier to stick to your low-fat diet at home.

The first step is to learn how to read nutrition labels. Use Figure 34.1 as your guide to a healthier heart.

A: Serving Size

Is your serving the same size as the one on the label? If you eat double the serving size listed, you need to double the nutrient and calorie values. If you eat one half the serving size shown here, cut the nutrient and calorie values in half.

B: Calories

Are you overweight? Cut back a little on calories! Look here to see how a serving of the food adds to your daily total. A 5' 4", 138-lb. active woman needs about 2,200 calories each day. A 5' 10", 174-lb. active man needs about 2,900. How about you?

"Shopping for a Healthy Heart," Information provided by the Norton Hospital Women's Pavilion Heart Center, © Norton Hospital, undated; reprinted with permission.

C: Total Carbohydrate

When you cut down on fat, you can eat more carbohydrates. Carbohydrates are in foods like bread, potatoes, fruits and vegetables. Choose these often! They give you nutrients and energy.

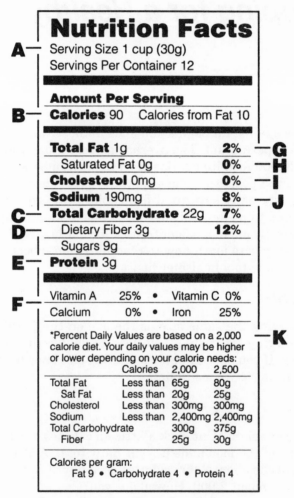

Source: American Heart Association

Figure 34.1.

D: Dietary Fiber

Grandmother called it "roughage," but her advice to eat more is still up-to-date! That goes for both soluble and insoluble kinds of dietary fiber. Fruits, vegetables, whole-grain foods, beans and peas are all good sources and can help reduce the risk of heart disease and cancer.

E: Protein

Most Americans get more protein than they need. Where there is animal protein, there is also fat and cholesterol. Eat small servings of lean meat, fish and poultry. Use skim or low-fat milk, yogurt and cheese. Try vegetable proteins like beans, grains and cereals.

F: Vitamins & Minerals

Your goal here is 100% of each for the day. Don't count on one food to do it all. Let a combination of foods add up to a winning score.

G: Total Fat

Aim low: Most people need to cut back on fat! Too much fat may contribute to heart disease and cancer. Try to limit your calories from fat. For a healthy heart, choose foods with a big difference between the total number of calories and the number of calories from fat.

H: Saturated Fat

A new kind of fat? No. Saturated fat is part of the total fat in food. It is listed separately because it's the key player in raising blood cholesterol and your risk of heart disease. Eat less!

I: Cholesterol

Too much cholesterol—a second cousin to fat—can lead to heart disease. Challenge yourself to eat less than 300 mg each day.

J: Sodium

You call it "salt," the label calls it "sodium." Either way, it may add up to high blood pressure in some people. So, keep your sodium intake low—2,400 to 3,000 mg or less each day.

K: Daily Value

Feel like you're drowning in numbers? Let the Daily Value be your guide. Daily Values are listed for people who eat 2,000 or 2,500 calories each day. If you eat more, your personal daily value may be higher than what's listed on the label. If you eat less, your personal daily value may be lower.

For fat, saturated fat, cholesterol and sodium, choose foods with a low "% Daily Value." For total carbohydrate, dietary fiber, vitamins and minerals, your daily value goal is to reach 100% of each. g = grams (about 28 = 1 ounce) mg = milligrams (1,000 mg = 1 g) For more information on making heart-healthy food choices, call The Women's Pavilion' Heart Center of The Norton Hospital—the area's first heart center designed for women—at 1-502-629-7000 or toll-free, outside Louisville, at 1-800-852-1770.

Chapter 35

Meal Planning: A Change of Heart

Getting serious about heart health may seem like a huge project. Because it means making basic changes in health and living habits, for many it is a major effort. But it doesn't have to be an overwhelming one. Some people find it easier to tackle only one habit at a time. If you smoke cigarettes and also eat a high-fat diet, for example, work on kicking the smoking habit first. Then, once you have gotten used to life without cigarettes, begin skimming the fat from your diet.

And remember: nobody's perfect. Nobody always eats the ideal diet or gets just the right amount of physical activity. Few smokers are able to swear off cigarettes without a slip or two along the way. The important thing is to follow a sensible, realistic plan that will gradually lessen your chances of developing heart disease, or help you to control it.

Women are taking a more active role in their own health care. We are asking more questions and we are seeking more self-help solutions. We are concerned not only about treatment, but also about the prevention of a wide range of health problems. Taking steps to control and prevent cardiovascular diseases is part of this growing movement to promote and protect personal health. The rewards of a healthy heart are well worth the effort.

Table 35.1 compares a higher fat diet, and a lower fat diet to give you a basic guide to begin "heart healthy" eating.

Table 35.2 is a guide to choosing low fat, low cholesterol foods.

Exerpted from *Heart Healthy Handbook for Women*, National Heart, Lung, and Blood Institute (NHLBI), NIH Publication No. 98-3654, revised August 1998.

Table 35.1. Example Meals for One Day

Higher-Fat Diet (37% Fat) | **Lower-Fat Diet (30% Fat)**

Breakfast
1 fried egg
2 slices white toast with
 1 teaspoon butter
1 cup orange juice

Breakfast
1 cup corn flakes with blueberries
1 cup 1% milk
1 slice rye toast with 1 teaspoon
 margarine
1 cup orange juice
black coffee or tea

Snack
1 doughnut

Snack
1 toasted pumpernickel bagel with 1
 teaspoon margarine

Lunch
1 grilled cheese (2 ounces)
 sandwich on white bread
2 oatmeal cookies
black coffee or tea

Lunch
1 tuna salad (3 ounces) sandwich on
 whole wheat bread with lettuce and
 tomato
1 graham cracker
tea with lemon

Snack
20 cheese cracker squares

Snack
1 crisp apple

Dinner
3 ounces fried hamburger with
 ketchup
1 baked potato with sour cream
3/4 cup steamed broccoli with
 1 teaspoon butter
1 cup whole milk
1 piece frosted marble cake

Dinner
3 ounces broiled lean ground beef with
 ketchup
1 baked potato with low fat plain yogurt
 and chives
1/4 cup steamed broccoli with 1 teaspoon margarine
tossed garden salad with 1 tablespoon
 oil and vinegar dressing
1 cup 1% milk
1 small piece homemade gingerbread
 with maraschino cherry and sprig of mint

Nutrient Analysis
Calories 2,000
Total fat (percent of calories) 37
Saturated fat (percent of calories) 19
Cholesterol 505 mgs

Nutrient Analysis
Calories 2,000
Total fat (percent of calories) 30
Saturated fat (percent of calories) 10
Cholesterol 186 mgs

Table 35.2. A Guide to Choosing Low Fat, Low-Cholesterol Foods

Variety is the spice of life. Choose foods every day from each of the following food groups. Choose different foods from within groups, especially foods low in saturated fat and cholesterol. As a guide, the recommended daily number of servings for adults is listed for each food group. But you'll have to decide on the number of servings you need to lose or maintain your weight. If you need help, ask a dietitian or your doctor.

Sources: Dietary Guidelines for Americans, U.S. Department of Agriculture/U.S. Department of Health and Human Services, 1995; Second Report of the Expert Panel on Detection, Evaluation, and Treatment of High Blood Cholesterol in Adults, NHLBI, 1993.

Breads, Cereals, Pasta, Rice

(6 to 11 servings daily; serving size is 1 slice bread, half a bun, or bagel, 1 ounce dry cereal, 1/2 cup cooked cereal, rice, or pasta)

Choose:
- Breads, like: whole wheat, pumpernickel, rye, and white; sandwich buns; dinner rolls; rice cakes
- Low fat crackers, like: matzah, pita; bagels; English muffins; bread sticks, rye, saltines, zwieback
- Hot cereals, most cold dry cereals
- Pasta, like: plain noodles, spaghetti, macaroni
- Any grain rice

Go Easy On:
- Store-bought pancakes, waffles, biscuits, muffins, cornbread

Decrease:
- Croissants, butter rolls, sweet rolls, Danish pastry, doughnuts
- Most snack crackers, like: cheese crackers, butter crackers, those made with saturated fats
- Granola-type cereals made with saturated fats
- Pasta and rice prepared with cream, butter, or cheese sauces, egg noodles

Table 35.2. A Guide to Choosing Low Fat, Low-Cholesterol Foods (continued)

Vegetables

(3 to 5 servings daily; serving is 1 cup leafy raw, cup cooked or chopped raw, 3/4 cup juice)

Choose:

• Fresh, frozen, canned, or dried vegetables

Decrease:

• Vegetables prepared in butter, cream, or sauce
• French fries

Fruits

(2 to 4 servings daily; serving is 1 piece, 1/2 cup diced, 3/4 cup fruit juice or cocktail)

Choose:

• Fresh, frozen, canned, or dried fruits

Go Easy On:

• Avocados and olives

Milk, Yogurt, and Cheese

(2 to 3 servings daily; 3 servings for women who are pregnant or breast feeding, and teenagers and young adults to age 24; serving size is 1 cup milk or yogurt; 1 ounce natural cheese, 11/2 ounce processed cheese)

Choose:

• Skim milk, 1% milk, skim-milk buttermilk, low fat evaporated or nonfat milk
• Nonfat or low fat yogurt and frozen yogurt
• Low fat and fat-free cheeses, string cheese, skim-milk buttermilk, low fat skim-milk, and fat-free cottage and ricotta cheese
• Nonfat sour cream

Table 35.2. A Guide to Choosing Low Fat, Low-Cholesterol Foods (continued)

Milk, Yogurt, and Cheese (continued)

Go Easy On:

- 2% milk
- Part-skim ricotta
- Part-skim or imitation hard cheeses, like: part-skim mozzarella
- "Light" cream cheese
- "Light" sour cream

Decrease:

- Whole milk, like: regular, evaporated, condensed
- Cream, half-and-half, most nondairy creamers and products, real or nondairy whipped cream
- Cream cheese, sour cream, ice cream, custard-style yogurt
- Whole-milk ricotta
- High-fat cheese, like: Neufchatel, Brie, Swiss, American, mozzarella, feta, cheddar, Muenster

Meat, Poultry, Fish, Dry Beans, Eggs, and Nuts

(2 to 3 servings daily)

Lean Meat, Poultry, Fish
(serving is 2-3 ounces of cooked lean meat poultry, or fish)

Choose:

- Lean cuts of meat with fat trimmed, like:
    Beef—round, sirloin, top loin, extra lean ground beef
    Lamb—leg-shank
    Pork—tenderloin, leg shank sirloin, top loin
    Veal—shoulder, ground, cutlet, sirloin
- Poultry without skin
- Fish, most shellfish

Table 35.2. A Guide to Choosing Low Fat, Low-Cholesterol Foods (continued)

Meat, Poultry, Fish, Dry Beans, Eggs, and Nuts (continued)

Lean Meat, Poultry, Fish (continued)

Go Easy On:
- Lean ground beef, flank steak
- Shrimp, abalone, squid

Decrease:
- Fatty cuts of meat like:

   Beef—brisket, regular ground, short ribs, chuck roast

   Lamb—rib, chops

   Pork—spareribs, blade roll or roast
- Goose, domestic duck
- Organ meats, like:

   liver

   kidney

   sweetbreads

   brain
- Sausage, bacon, frankfurters, regular luncheon meats
- Caviar, roe

Dry Beans and Peas
(serving is 1/2 cup tofu or cooked dry peas or beans—1/2 cup cooked dry beans or 2 Tbsp of peanut butter or 1/3 cup of nuts counts as 1 ounce of lean meat)

Choose:
- Dried peas and beans, like: split peas, black-eyed peas, chick peas, kidney beans, navy beans, lentils, soybeans, soybean curd (tofu)

Go Easy On:
- Refried beans (read food label for fat content)

Table 35.2. A Guide to Choosing Low Fat, Low-Cholesterol Foods (continued)

Meat, Poultry, Fish, Dry Beans, Eggs, and Nuts (continued)

Eggs
(no more than 4 egg yolks a week)

Choose:
- Egg whites
- Cholesterol-free egg substitutes

Decrease:
- Egg yolks
- Whole eggs

Nuts
(serving is 1/3 CUP)

Go Easy On:
- Nuts and seeds
- Peanut butter

Fats, Oils, and Sweets
(use sparingly)

Fats and Oils

Choose:
- Unsaturated vegetable oils like: corn, olive, peanut, rapeseed (canola oil), safflower, sesame, soybean
- Margarine or shortening made with unsaturated fats listed above: diet and tub
- Low fat and fat-free mayonnaise, low fat and fat-free salad dressings made with unsaturated fats listed above

Decrease:
- Butter, coconut oil, palm kernel oil, palm oil, lard, bacon fat
- Stick margarine or shortening made with saturated fats listed above
- Dressings made with egg yolk, such as hollandaise sauce and Caesar salad dressing
- Regular salad dressing and mayonnaise

Table 35.2. A Guide to Choosing Low Fat, Low-Cholesterol Foods (continued)

Fats, Oils, and Sweets (continued)

Sweets and Snacks
(Remember: fat-free and low fat choices may be high in calories)

Choose:

- Nonfat and low fat frozen desserts, like: sherbet, sorbet, Italian ice, frozen yogurt, popsicles
- Fat-free cakes and cookies
- Low fat cakes, like: angel food cake
- Low fat cookies, like: fig bars, gingersnaps
- Low fat candy, like: jelly beans, hard candy
- Low fat snacks, like: plain popcorn, pretzels, graham crackers
- Nonfat beverages, like: carbonated drinks, juices, tea, coffee

Go Easy On:

- Frozen desserts, like: ice milk
- Homemade cakes, cookies, and pies using unsaturated oils sparingly
- Fruit crisps and cobblers
- Potato and corn chips prepared with unsaturated vegetable oil

Decrease:

- High-fat frozen desserts, like: ice cream, frozen tofu
- High-fat cakes, like: most store-bought pound, and frosted cakes
- Regular pies and cookies
- Most candy, like: chocolate bars
- Potato and corn chips prepared with saturated fat
- Buttered popcorn
- High-fat beverages, like: frappes, milkshakes, floats, eggnogs

Table 35.2. A Guide to Choosing Low Fat, Low-Cholesterol Foods (continued)

Label Ingredients

(Choose foods lower in fat saturated fat, or cholesterol, go easy on products that list first any fat oil, or ingredients higher in saturated fat or cholesterol. Choose more often those products that contain ingredients lower in saturated fat or cholesterol.)

Choose:

- Ingredients Lower in Saturated Fat or Cholesterol: carob, cocoa; oils, like: corn, cottonseed, olive, safflower, sesame, soybean, or sunflower; nonfat dry milk, nonfat dry milk solids, skim milk

Decrease:

- Sources of Saturated Fat and Cholesterol: animal fat, bacon fat, beef fat, butter, chicken fat, cocoa butter, coconut, coconut oil, cream, egg and egg-yolk solids, ham fat, hardened fat or oil, hydrogenated vegetable oil, lamb fat, lard, meat fat, palm kernel oil, palm oil, pork fat, turkey fat, coconut, palm, or palm kernel oil, vegetable shortening, whole-milk solids

Chapter 36

Recipes for a Healthy Heart

These recipes come from various ethnic groups and include soups, entrees, side dishes, and desserts. They're full of taste but lower in fat, cholesterol, and sodium.

Minestrone

A cholesterol free classic Italian vegetable soup brimming with fiber-rich beans, peas, and carrots.

1/4 C	olive oil
1 clove	garlic, minced or 1/8 tsp garlic powder
1 1/3 C	coarsely chopped onion
1 1/2 C	coarsely chopped celery and leaves
1 Tbsp	chopped fresh parsley
1 C	sliced carrots, fresh or frozen
4 3/4 C	shredded cabbage
1 can (1 lb.)	tomatoes, cut up
1 C	canned red kidney beans, drained and rinsed
1 1/2 C	frozen peas
1 1/2 C	green beans

Exerpted from *Heart Healthy Handbook for Women*, National Heart, Lung, and Blood Institute (NHLBI), NIH Publication No. 98-3654, revised August 1998.

1 can (6 oz)	tomato paste
dash	hot sauce
11 C	water
2 C	uncooked, broken spaghetti

1. Heat oil in a 4-quart saucepan.

2. Add garlic, onion, and celery and sauté about 5 minutes.

3. Add all remaining ingredients except spaghetti, and stir until ingredients are well mixed.

4. Bring to a boil. Reduce heat, cover, and simmer about 45 minutes or until vegetables are tender.

5. Add uncooked spaghetti and simmer 2-3 minutes only.

Yield: 16 servings

Serving size: 1 cup

Each serving provides: 153 calories; 4 g total fat; 0 mg cholesterol; 191 mg sodium.

Rockport Fish Chowder

Low fat milk and clam juice are the secrets to the lower fat and saturated fat content of this satisfying supper soup.

2 Tbsp	vegetable oil
3/4 C	coarsely chopped onion
1 1/2 C	coarsely chopped celery
1 C	sliced carrots
2 C	potatoes, raw, peeled and cubed
1/4 tsp	thyme
1/2 tsp	paprika
2 C	bottled clam juice
8	whole peppercorns
1	bay leaf
1 lb.	fresh or frozen (thawed) cod or haddock fillets, cut into 3/4-inch cubes
1/4 C	flour

3 C	low fat (1%) milk
1 Tbsp	fresh parsley, chopped

1. Heat oil in a large saucepan. Add onion and celery and sauté about 3 minutes.

2. Add carrots, potatoes, thyme, paprika, and clam broth. Wrap peppercorns and bay leaves in cheese cloth. Add to pot. Bring to a boil, reduce heat, and simmer 15 minutes.

3. Add fish and simmer an additional 15 minutes, or until fish flakes easily and is opaque.

4. Remove fish and vegetables; break fish into chunks. Bring broth to a boil and continue boiling until volume is reduced to 1 cup. Remove bay leaves and peppercorns.

5. Shake flour and 1/2 cup low fat (1%) milk in a container with a tight-fitting lid until smooth. Add to broth in saucepan with remaining milk. Cook over medium heat, stirring constantly, until mixture boils and is thickened.

6. Return vegetables and fish chunks to stock and heat thoroughly. Serve hot, sprinkled with chopped parsley.

Yield: 8 servings

Serving size: 1 cup each

Each serving provides: 186 calories; 6 g total fat; 1 g saturated fat, 34 mg cholesterol, 302 mg sodium.

Baked Trout

Try baking this fish with only a small amount of oil.

2 lb.	trout fillet, cut into 6 pieces (or use any kind of fish)
3 Tbsp	lime juice (about 2 limes)
1	medium tomato, chopped
1/2	medium onion, chopped
3 Tbsp	cilantro, chopped
1/2 tsp	olive oil
1/4 tsp	black pepper
1/4 tsp	salt

1/4 tsp	red pepper (optional)

1. Preheat oven to 350° F

2. Rinse fish and pat dry. Place in baking dish.

3. In a separate dish, mix remaining ingredients together and pour over fish.

4. Bake for 15-20 minutes or until fork-tender.

Yields: 6 servings

Serving size: 1 piece

Each serving provides: 230 calories; 9 g total fat; 2 g saturated fat; 58 mg cholesterol; 162 mg sodium.

Mediterranean Baked Fish

This dish is baked and flavored with a Mediterranean-style tomato, onion, and garlic sauce to make it lower in fat and salt.

2 tsp	olive oil
1	large onion, sliced
1 can	(16 oz) whole tomatoes, drained (reserve juice) and coarsely chopped
1	bay leaf
1	clove garlic, minced
1 C	dry white wine
1/2 C	reserved tomato juice from canned tomatoes
1/4 C	lemon juice
1/4 C	orange juice
1 Tbsp	fresh grated orange peel
1 tsp	fennel seeds, crushed
1/2 tsp	dried oregano, crushed
1/2 tsp	dried thyme, crushed
1/2 tsp	dried basil, crushed
to taste	black pepper
1 lb.	fish fillets (sole, flounder, or sea perch)

1. Heat oil in large nonstick skillet. Add onion, and sauté over moderate heat 5 minutes or until soft.

2. Add all remaining ingredients except fish.

3. Stir well and simmer 30 minutes, uncovered.

4. Arrange fish in 10 x 6-inch baking dish; cover with sauce.

5. Bake, uncovered, at 375° F about 15 minutes or until fish flakes easily. Remove bay leaf before serving.

Yield: 4 servings

Serving size: 4 oz fillet with sauce

Each serving provides: 177 calories; 4 g total fat; 1 g saturated fat 56 mg cholesterol; 281 mg sodium.

Spaghetti with Turkey Meat Sauce

Using nonstick cooking spray, ground turkey, and no added salt helps to make this classic dish heart-healthy.

as needed	nonstick cooking spray
1 lb.	ground turkey
1 can	(28 oz) tomatoes, cut up
1 C	finely chopped green pepper
1 C	finely chopped onion
2 cloves	garlic, minced
1 tsp	dried oregano, crushed
1 tsp	black pepper
1 lb.	spaghetti, uncooked

1. Spray a large skillet with nonstick spray coating. Preheat over high heat.

2. Add turkey; cook, stirring occasionally, for 5 minutes. Drain fat and discard.

3. Stir in tomatoes with their juice, green pepper, onion, garlic, oregano, and black pepper. Bring to a boil; reduce heat, Simmer covered for 15 minutes, stirring occasionally. Remove cover; simmer for 15 minutes more. (If you like a creamier sauce, give sauce a whirl in your blender or food processor.)

4. Meanwhile, cook spaghetti in unsalted water. Drain well.

5. Serve sauce over spaghetti.

Yield: 6 servings

Serving size: 5 oz sauce and 9 oz spaghetti

Each serving provides: 330 calories; 5 g total fat; 1 g saturated fat; 60 mg cholesterol; 280 mg sodium.

Chicken Orientale

With no added salt and very little oil in the marinade, these broiled or grilled kabobs made with skinless chicken breasts are lower in saturated fat, cholesterol, and sodium.

8	boneless, skinless chicken breasts
8	fresh mushrooms
to taste	black pepper
8	parboiled whole white onions
2	oranges, quartered
8	canned pineapple chunks
8	cherry tomatoes
1	6 oz can frozen, concentrated apple juice, thawed
1 C	dry white wine
2 Tbsp	soy sauce, low sodium
dash	ground ginger
2 Tbsp	vinegar
1/4 C	vegetable oil

1. Sprinkle chicken breasts with pepper.

2. Thread 8 skewers as follows: chicken, mushroom, chicken, onion, chicken, orange quarter, chicken, pineapple chunk, cherry tomato.

3. Place kabobs in shallow pan.

4. Combine remaining ingredients and save 1/2 cup in another bowl; spoon the rest over kabobs. Marinate in refrigerator at least 1 hour.

5. Drain. Broil 6 inches from heat, 15 minutes on each side, brushing with reserved marinade every 5 minutes. Discard any leftover marinade.

Yield: 8 servings

Serving size: 1/2 chicken breast kabob

Each serving provides: 359 calories; 11 g total fat 2 g saturated fat; 66 mg cholesterol; 226 mg sodium.

Chicken and Rice

Skinned chicken makes this dish lower in saturated fat and calories.

6	chicken pieces (legs and breasts), skinned
2 tsp	vegetable oil
4 C	water
2	tomatoes, chopped
1/2 C	green pepper, chopped
1/4 C	red pepper, chopped
1/4 C	celery, diced
1	medium carrot, grated
1/4 C	corn, frozen
1/2 C	onion, chopped
1/4 C	fresh cilantro, chopped
2 cloves	garlic, chopped fine
1/8 tsp	salt
1/8 tsp	pepper
2 C	rice
1/2 C	peas, frozen
2 ounces	Spanish olives
1/4 C	raisins

1. In a large pot, brown chicken pieces in oil.

2. Add water, tomatoes, green and red peppers, celery, carrots, corn, onion, cilantro, garlic, salt, and pepper. Cover and cook over medium heat for 20-30 minutes or until chicken is done.

3. Remove chicken from the pot and place in the refrigerator. Add rice, peas, and olives to the pot. Cover pot and cook over low heat for about 20 minutes, until rice is cooked.

4. Add chicken and raisins and cook for another 8 minutes.

Yield: 6 servings

Serving size: 1 cup rice and 1 piece chicken

Each serving provides: 448 calories; 7 g total fat; 2 g saturated fat; 49 mg cholesterol; 352 mg sodium.

Grilled Chicken with Green Chile Sauce

The secret to this dish is marinating the meat, which makes it tender without adding a lot of fat.

4	skinless, boneless chicken breasts
1/4 C	olive oil
juice of 2	limes
1/4 tsp	oregano
1/2 tsp	black pepper
1/4 C	water
10-12	tomatillos, husks removed and cut in half
1/2	medium onion, quartered
2 cloves	garlic, finely chopped
2	serrano or jalapeno peppers
2 Tbsp	cilantro, chopped
1/4 tsp	salt
1/4 C	low fat sour cream

1. Combine the oil, juice from 1 lime, oregano, and black pepper in a shallow glass baking dish. Stir. Place the chicken breasts in the baking dish and turn to coat each side. Cover the dish and refrigerate for at least several hours or overnight. Turn the chicken periodically to marinate chicken on both sides.

2. Put water, tomatillos, and onion into a saucepan. Bring to a gentle boil and cook uncovered for 10 minutes or until the tomatillos are tender. In a blender, place the cooked onion, tomatillos, and any remaining water. Add the garlic, peppers,

cilantro, salt, and the remaining lime juice. Blend until all the ingredients are smooth. Place the sauce in a bowl and refrigerate.

3. Place the chicken breast on a hot grill and cook until done. Place the chicken on a serving platter.

4. Spoon a tablespoon of low fat sour cream over the chicken breast. Pour the sauce over the sour cream.

Yield: 4 servings

Serving size: 1 breast

Each serving provides: 192 calories; 5 g total fat; 2 g saturated fat; 71 mg cholesterol; 220 mg sodium.

Baked Pork Chops

These spicy and moist pork chops are made with no added fat, egg whites, evaporated skim milk, and a lively herb mixture that contains no salt.

6	lean center-cut pork chops, 1/3-inch thick
1	egg white
1 C	evaporated skim milk
3/4 C	cornflake crumbs
1/4 C	fine dry bread crumbs
4 tsp	paprika
2 tsp	oregano
1/4 tsp	chili powder
1/2 tsp	garlic powder
1/2 tsp	black pepper
1/8 tsp	cayenne pepper
1/8 tsp	dry mustard
1/2 tsp	salt
as needed	nonstick spray coating

1. Trim all fat from chops.

2. Beat egg white with evaporated skim milk. Place chops in milk mixture and let stand for 5 minutes, turning chops once.

3. Meanwhile, mix together cornflake crumbs, bread crumbs, spices, and salt.

4. Spray a 9x13-inch baking pan with nonstick spray coating.

5. Remove chops from milk mixture. Coat thoroughly with crumb mixture.

6. Place chops in pan and bake in 375° F oven for 20 minutes. Turn chops and bake 15 minutes longer or till no pink remains.

Note: If desired, substitute skinless, boneless chicken, turkey parts, or fish for pork chops and bake for 20 minutes.

Yield: 6 servings
Serving size: 1 pork chop
Each serving provides: 186 calories; 5 g total fat; 2 g saturated fat; 31 mg cholesterol; 393 mg sodium.

Bavarian Beef

This classic German stew is made with lean trimmed beef stew meat and cabbage.

1 1/4 lb.	lean beef stew meat (trimmed of fat), cut in 1-inch pieces
1 Tbsp	vegetable oil
1	large onion, thinly sliced
1 1/2 C	water
1/4 tsp	caraway seeds
1/2 tsp	salt
1/8 tsp	black pepper
1	bay leaf
1/4 C	white vinegar
1 Tbsp	sugar
1/2	small head red cabbage, cut into 4 wedges
1/4 C	crushed gingersnaps

1. Brown meat in oil in a heavy skillet. Remove meat and sauté onion in remaining oil until golden. Return meat to skillet.

Add water, caraway seeds, salt, pepper, and bay leaf. Bring to a boil. Reduce heat, cover, and simmer 1 1/4 hours.

2. Add vinegar and sugar; stir. Place cabbage on top of meat. Cover and simmer 45 minutes more.

3. Arrange meat and cabbage on a platter and keep warm.

4. Strain drippings and skim off fat. Add enough water to drippings to yield 1 cup of liquid. Return to skillet with gingersnap crumbs. Cook and stir until thickened and mixture boils. Serve with meat and vegetables.

Yield: 5 servings

Serving size: 5 oz

Each serving provides: 244 calories; 11 g total fat; 3 g saturated fat; 56 mg cholesterol; 323 mg sodium.

New Orleans Red Beans

This vegetarian main dish is cholesterol free, virtually fat free, and chock full of vegetables.

1 lb.	dry red beans
2 qt	water
1 1/2 C	chopped onion
1 C	chopped celery
4	bay leaves
1 C	chopped green pepper
3 Tbsp	chopped garlic
3 Tbsp	chopped parsley
2 tsp	dried thyme, crushed
1 tsp	salt
1 tsp	black pepper

1. Pick through beans to remove bad beans; rinse thoroughly.

2. In a large pot combine beans, water, onion, celery, and bay leaves. Bring to a boil; reduce heat. Cover and cook over low heat for about 1 1/2 hours or until beans are tender. Stir. Mash beans against side of pan.

3. Add green pepper, garlic, parsley, thyme, salt, and black pepper. Cook uncovered, over low heat till creamy, about 30 minutes. Remove bay leaves.

4. Serve with hot cooked brown rice, if desired.

Yield: 8 servings

Serving size: 1 1/4 cup

Each serving provides: 171 calories; less than 1 g total fat; less than 1 g saturated fat; 0 cholesterol; 285 mg sodium.

Sweet & Sour Seashells

Draining the marinade before serving keeps the fat and sodium low in this cold pasta salad.

1 lb.	uncooked small seashell macaroni (9 cups cooked)
2 Tbsp	vegetable oil
1/4 C	sugar
1/2 C	cider vinegar
1/2 C	wine vinegar
1/2 C	water
3 Tbsp	prepared mustard
to taste	black pepper
2 oz jar	sliced pimentos
2	small cucumbers
2	small onions thinly sliced
18	lettuce leaves

1. Cook macaroni in unsalted water, drain, rinse with cold water, and drain again. Stir in oil.

2. Transfer to 4-quart bowl. Place sugar, vinegars, water, prepared mustard, pepper, and pimento in blender. Process at low speed 15-20 seconds, or just enough so flecks of pimento can be seen. Pour over macaroni.

3. Score cucumber peel with fork tines. Cut cucumber in half lengthwise, then slice thinly. Add to pasta with onion slices. Toss well.

4. Marinate, covered, in refrigerator 24 hours. Stir occasionally.

5. Drain and serve on lettuce.

Yield: 18 servings

Serving size: 1/2 cup

Each serving provides: 149 calories; 2 g total fat; less than 1 g saturated fat; 0 mg cholesterol; 33 mg sodium.

Vegetables with a Touch of Lemon

Lemon juice, herbs, and a small amount of oil make this sauce as tasty as it is healthy.

1/2	small head cauliflower, cut into florets
2 C	broccoli, cut into florets
2 Tbsp	lemon juice
1 Tbsp	olive oil
1 clove	garlic, minced
2 tsp	fresh parsley, chopped

1. Steam broccoli and cauliflower until tender (about 10 minutes).

2. In a small saucepan, mix the lemon juice, oil, and garlic, and cook over low heat for 2 or 3 minutes.

3. Put the vegetables in a serving dish. Pour the lemon sauce over the vegetables. Garnish with parsley.

Yield: 6 servings

Serving size: 1/2 C

Each serving provides: 22 calories; 2 g total fat; less than 1 g saturated fat; 0 mg cholesterol; 7 mg sodium.

Garlic Mashed Potatoes

No added fat or salt is used or needed in this tasty potato dish.

1 lb.	(about 2 large) potatoes, peeled and quartered
2 C	skim milk
2 large	cloves garlic, chopped

273

1/2 tsp   white pepper

1. Cook potatoes, covered, in a small amount of boiling water for 20-25 minutes or until tender. Remove from heat. Drain and recover.

2. Meanwhile, in a small saucepan over low heat, cook garlic in milk until garlic is soft, about 30 minutes.

3. Add milk-garlic mixture and white pepper to potatoes. Beat with an electric mixer on low speed or mash with a potato masher until smooth.

Microwave Directions

Scrub potatoes, pat dry, and prick with a fork. On a plate, cook potatoes, uncovered, on 100% power (high) until tender, about 12 minutes, turning potatoes over once. Let stand 5 minutes. Peel and quarter. Meanwhile, in a 4-cup glass measuring cup, combine milk and garlic. Cook, uncovered, on 50% power (medium) until garlic is soft, about 4 minutes. Continue as directed above.

Yield: 4 servings

Serving size: 3/4 cup

Each serving provides: 141 calories; less than 1 g total fat; less than 1 g saturated fat; 2 mg cholesterol; 70 mg sodium.

Crunchy Pumpkin Pie

This pie uses only a small amount of oil in the crust and skim milk in the filling to make it heart-healthy.

For the Pie Crust

1 C	quick cooking oats
1/4 C	whole wheat flour
1/4 C	ground almonds
2 Tbsp	brown sugar
1/4 tsp	salt
3 Tbsp	vegetable oil
1 Tbsp	water

For the Pie Filling

1/4 C	packed brown sugar
1/2 tsp	ground cinnamon
1/4 tsp	ground nutmeg
1/4 tsp	salt
1	egg, beaten
4 tsp	vanilla
1 C	canned pumpkin
2/3 C	evaporated skim milk

1. Preheat oven to 425° F.

2. Mix oats, flour, almonds, sugar, and salt together in small mixing bowl.

3. Blend oil and water together in measuring cup with fork or small wire whisk until emulsified.

4. Add oil mixture to dry ingredients and mix well. If needed, add small amount of water to hold mixture together.

5. Press into a 9-inch pie pan and bake for 8-10 minutes, or until light brown.

6. Turn down oven to 350° F.

7. Mix sugar, cinnamon, nutmeg, and salt together in a bowl.

8. Add eggs and vanilla and mix to blend ingredients.

9. Add pumpkin and milk and stir to combine.

10. Pour into prepared pie shells.

11. Bake 45 minutes at 350° F or until knife inserted near center comes out clean.

Yield: 9 servings

Serving size: 1/9 of a 9-inch pie

Each serving provides: 177 calories; 8 g total fat; 1 g saturated fat; 24 mg cholesterol; 153 mg sodium.

Rice Pudding

This delicious dessert reduces the fat and calories by using skim instead of whole milk.

6 C	water
2	cinnamon sticks
1 C	rice
3 C	skim milk
2/3 C	sugar
1/2 tsp	salt

1. Put the water and cinnamon sticks into a medium saucepan. Bring to a boil.

2. Stir in rice. Cook on low heat for 30 minutes until rice is soft and water has evaporated.

3. Add skim milk, sugar, and salt. Cook for another 15 minutes until it thickens.

Yield: 5 servings

Serving size: 1/2 cup

Each serving provides: 372 calories; less than 1 g total fat; less than 1 g saturated fat; 3 mg cholesterol; 366 mg sodium.

Winter Crisp

Only 1 tablespoon of margarine is used to make the crumb topping of this tart and tangy fruit dessert that is cholesterol free and low in sodium.

For the Filling

1/2 C	sugar
3 Tbsp	all-purpose flour
1 tsp	lemon peel, grated
1/4 tsp	lemon juice
5 C	apples, unpeeled, sliced
1 C	cranberries

For the Topping

1/3 C	rolled oats
1/3 C	brown sugar, packed
1/4 C	whole wheat flour
2 tsp	ground cinnamon
1 Tbsp	soft margarine, melted

1. To prepare filling, in a medium bowl combine sugar, flour, and lemon peel; mix well. Add lemon juice, apples, and cranberries; stir to mix. Spoon into a 6-cup baking dish.

2. To prepare topping, in a small bowl, combine oats, brown sugar, flour, and cinnamon. Add melted margarine; stir to mix.

3. Sprinkle topping over filling. Bake in a 375° F oven for approximately 40-50 minutes or until filling is bubbly and top is brown. Serve warm or at room temperature.

Note: For a summertime crisp, prepare as directed but substitute 4 cups fresh or unsweetened frozen (thawed) peaches and 3 cups fresh or unsweetened frozen (unthawed) blueberries for apples and cranberries. If frozen, thaw peaches completely (do not drain). Do not thaw blueberries before mixing or they will be crushed.

Yield: 6 servings

Serving size: 1 3/4-inch by 2-inch piece

Each serving provides: 284 calories; 6 g total fat; 1 g saturated fat; 0 mg cholesterol; 56 mg sodium.

Part Six

Additional Help and Information

Chapter 37

Glossary of Important Terms

ACE inhibitor: Stops production of a chemical that makes blood vessels narrow and is used for high blood pressure and heart muscle that has been damaged.

aspirin: Helps prevent heart attacks when taken regularly in a low dose on a doctor's orders.

atherosclerosis: The gradual build up of fatty substances in blood vessels, which become narrowed and less flexible, until blood does not flow easily through them or is completely blocked.

beta-blocker: Reduces how hard the heart must work and is used for high blood pressure, chest pain, and to prevent a repeat heart attack.

blood cholesterol-lowering agents: HMG CoA reductase inhibitors (or "statins"), nicotinic acid, bile acid sequestrants, fibric acid derivatives, and probucol.

calcium-channel blocker: Relaxes blood vessels; used for high blood pressure and chest pain.

Compiled from "Hormone Replacement Therapy and Heart Disease: The PEPI Trial," National Heart, Lung, and Blood Institute (NHLBI), NIH Publication No. 95-3277, August 1995; and from *Heart Healthy Handbook for Women*, National Heart, Lung, and Blood Institute (NHLBI), NIH Publication No. 98-3654, revised August 1998.

cardiovascular disease: A disease of the heart or blood vessels. Cardiovascular diseases include heart disease, heart attack, stroke, and atherosclerosis.

cholesterol: A waxy substance produced by the body and needed for many functions, such as helping to make cell membranes and some hormones.

clinical trial: A scientific test that compares different treatments. It often uses a placebo for comparison and may be double-blind, which means that neither participants nor researchers and doctors know who is on what treatment.

combined hormone therapy: When estrogen is taken with progestin.

continuous hormone therapy: Talking hormones daily.

coronary angiography (or arteriography): Displays blood flow problems and blockages. A fine, flexible tube (or "catheter") is threaded through an artery of an arm or leg up into the heart. A fluid that shows up on x-ray is then injected, and the heart and blood vessels are filmed as the heart pumps. The picture is called an angiogram or arteriogram.

coronary angioplasty: Also called "balloon" angioplasty. A fine tube is threaded through an artery to the narrowed heart vessel, where a tiny balloon at its tip is inflated. The balloon flattens the buildup and stretches the artery, improving blood flow. It is then deflated and removed, along with the tube.

coronary artery bypass graft surgery: Also known as "bypass surgery." A piece of blood vessel is taken from the leg or chest and is stitched onto the narrowed heart artery, making a bypass around the blockage. Sometimes, more than one bypass is needed.

Bypass surgery is used when blockages in an artery can't be reached by, or are too long or hard for, angioplasty. A bypass requires about 1 week in the hospital and several weeks of recuperation at home.

coronary heart disease: A disease of the blood vessels of the heart that can cause heart attacks.

cyclic hormone therapy: Taking hormones only on certain days.

diabetes: High blood sugar, a serious disorder. The risk of death from heart disease is about three times higher for women with diabetes than for those without the condition. After age 45, about twice as many women as men develop diabetes. The condition can often be controlled or prevented with lifestyle changes, such as weight loss and physical activity.

digitalis: Makes the heart contract harder and is used when the heart's pumping function has been weakened; it also slows some fast heart rhythms.

diuretic: Decreases fluid in the body and is used for high blood pressure.

echocardiography: Converts sound waves, bounced off the heart, into images that show heart size, shape, and movement. The sound waves also can be used to see how much blood is pumped out by the heart when it contracts.

electrocardiogram (ECG or EKG): Makes a graphic record of the heart's electrical activity as it beats. This can show abnormal heartbeats, muscle damage, blood flow problems, and heart enlargement.

endometrial biopsy: Removal of some cells of the lining of the uterus for examination.

endometrial hyperplasia: Abnormal growth of cells that line the uterus. If severe, it may develop into cancer.

endometrium: Lining of the uterus.

estrogen: Hormone produced by the ovaries until menopause and important in helping to regulate the menstrual cycle. It is now believed to help reduce the risk of heart disease.

estrogen replacement therapy: Hormone replacement therapy that uses only estrogen.

HDL—high-density lipoprotein: Often called the "good" cholesterol because it helps remove cholesterol from the blood.

HRT—hormone replacement therapy: Estrogen is taken alone or with progestin.

hypertension—high blood pressure: A condition in which blood pressure is at or above 140/90 mm Hg. It usually produces no symptoms but if not treated can result in serious health problems. It is a risk factor for heart disease and stroke.

hysterectomy: Surgical removal of the uterus. A woman who has had her uterus removed but not her ovaries does not become menopausal until her ovaries stop producing hormones.

lipids: Fatty substances, including cholesterol and triglycerides. Lipids are present in blood and tissues.

mammogram: X-ray of the breast, also called mammography.

menopause: The end of menstruation, when the ovaries stop producing estrogen, progesterone, and other hormones. "Natural menopause" applies to women who are usually approximately age 45-54 and who have gone 12 months without a period, including no spotting; "surgical menopause" refers to women who have had both ovaries removed.

micronized progesterone: A natural form of the hormone progesterone.

nitrate (including nitroglycerine): Relaxes blood vessels and alleviates chest pain.

nuclear scan: Assesses heart muscle contraction as blood flows through the heart. A small amount of radioactive material is injected into a vein, usually in the arm, and a scanning camera then records how much is taken up by the heart muscle.

PEPI—Postmenopausal Estrogen/Progestin Interventions Trial: Conducted at seven American clinical centers. PEPI is the first major clinical trial to examine the effects of estrogen and progestin replacement therapies on heart disease risk factors in postmenopausal women.

placebo: A substance that looks like a drug but has no biological effect.

post menopausal: A woman who has gone through menopause.

progesterone/progestin: Two words often used interchangeably. Progesterone is a hormone produced by the ovaries until menopause; it is important in controlling the growth of cells lining the uterus. Progestin is a synthetic form of progesterone.

progestin: A synthetic form of progesterone.

regimen: Schedule of medication.

stress test (or treadmill test or exercise ECG): Records the ECG during exercise, usually on a treadmill or exercise bicycle. Some heart problems show up only when more effort is asked of the heart, as happens during increased activity. So the exercise ECG may be done even if the resting ECG is normal.

Other exercise tests may be done with an ECG or a nuclear scan to assess heart muscle contraction or blood flow in the heart.

Older women may not be able to exercise due to arthritis or another condition. For them, a stress test can be done without exercise by using a drug that increases blood flow.

stroke: Damage to the brain resulting from blockage of blood flow to the brain or from hemorrhage (bleeding) of blood into the brain.

triglyceride: A type of lipid carried through the blood to tissues. Most of the body's fat tissue is in the form of triglycerides, stored for use as energy.

Chapter 38

Resources for a Healthy Heart

General Resources for Women's Heart Health

The American Dietetic Association
216 W. Jackson Blvd.
Suite 800
Chicago, IL 60606-6995
Phone: (312) 899-0040
Fax: (312) 899-1979

American Heart Association (AHA)
National Center
7320 Greenville Avenue
Dallas, TX 75231
Toll-free: (800) AHA-USA1
Website: http://www.amhrt.org/

Contact the national office or your local AHA affiliate for a list of publications on heart health. Single copies of most publications are free.

Information in this chapter was compiled from *Heart Healthy Handbook for Women*, National Heart, Lung, and Blood Institute (NHLBI), NIH Publication No. 98-3654, revised August 1998; and *Diet and Nutrition Materials for Consumers*, Weight-Control Information Network (WIN), August 1997; and *Sensible Nutrition Resource List for Consumers*, U.S. Department of Agriculture, August 1998.

American Institute of Nutrition
American Society for Clinical Nutrition, Inc.
9650 Rockville Pike
Bethesda, MD 20814-3998
Phone: (301) 530-7050
E-mail: meyersp@ain.faseb.org
Website: http://www.faseb.org/ain/

Consumer Information Center (CIC)
Catalog
Pueblo, CO 81009
Phone: (719) 948-4000
Website: http://www.pueblo.gsa.gov

CIC has free or low-cost consumer booklets from more than 40 Federal departments and agencies, including the U.S. Department of Agriculture and the U.S. Food and Drug Administration. Topics include the Dietary Guidelines for Americans, the food labels, and other health issues. For a catalog, write or call the CIC. The catalog and many of the publications also are available on the Internet.

National Cancer Institute (NCI)
Office of Cancer Communications
Bldg. 31, Room 1OA24
9000 Rockville Pike
Bethesda, MD 20892
Toll-free: (800) 4-CANCER
Phone: (301) 496-5583
Website: http://www.nci.nih.gov/

Provides free publications on how to stop smoking and many other cancer-related topics.

National Heart, Lung, and Blood Institute (NHLBI)
Information Center
PO. Box 30105
Bethesda, MD 20824-0105
Toll-free: (800) 575-WELL
Phone: (301) 251-1222
Website: http://www.nhibi.nih.gov

Call the 800 number for information about the prevention and control of high blood pressure and high blood cholesterol. Write for a list of free or low-cost publications on all aspects of heart health.

National Institute on Aging (NIA)
Information Center
PO. Box 8057
Gaithersburg, MD 20898-8057
Toll-free: (800) 222-2225
TTY: (800) 222-4225 (for hearing impaired)
Website: http://www.nih.gov/nia

Provides information on a wide range of topics related to health and aging, including physical activities for older persons.

Weight-control Information Network
1 Win Way
Bethesda, MD 20892-3665
301-984-7378
800-WIN-8098
Fax: 301-984-7196
E-mail: win@info.niddk.nih.gov

Internet: http://www.niddk.nih.gov/health/nutrit/win.htm

Cookbooks *(in alphabetical order by title)*

American Heart Association Cookbook, 5th edition
M. Winston
New York, NY: Random House, 1991, 643 p.
Random House, 1540 Broadway, New York, NY 10036; (212) 782-9000; (212) 302-7985 fax

American Medical Association Family Health Cookbook
Melanie Barnard and Brooke Dojny
New York, NY: Pocket Books, 1997, 513 p.
Pocket Books, 1230 Avenue of the Americas, New York, NY 10020; (212) 698-7000

Cooking for Few: A Guide to Easy Cooking for One or Two
Australia: National Heart Foundation of Australia, 1991, 116 p.
National Heart Foundation of Australia, Cnr. Dennison St. & Geils Court, Deakin, A.C.T. 2606

Free and Equal Dessert Cookbook
C. Kruppa
Chicago, IL: Surrey Books, 1992, 167 p.
Surrey Books, 230 East Ohio Street, Suite 120, Chicago, IL 60611; (800) 326-4430 or (312) 751-7330

The Guilt-Free Comfort Food Cookbook
Georgia Kostas with Robert A. Barnett
Nashville: T. Nelson Publishers, 1996, 301 p.
T. Nelson Publishers, 501 Nelson Pl., Nashville, TN 37214; (615) 889-9000

Healthy Weeknight Meals in Minutes
David Joachim (editor)
Emmaus, PA: Rodale Press, Inc., 1997, 312 p.
Rodale Press, Inc., 33 E. Minor St., Emmaus, PA 18098; (610) 967-8154

Lowfat Cooking for Dummies
Lynn Fischer
Foster City, CA: IDG Books Worldwide, Inc., 1997, 408 p.
IDG Books Worldwide, Inc., 919 E. Hillsdale Blvd., Suite 400, Foster City, CA 94404; (650) 655-3000

Low-Fat & Luscious: Breakfasts, Snacks, Main Dishes, Side Dishes, Desserts
Kristi Fuller (editor)
Des Moines, IA: Meredith Corp., 1996, 160 p.
Meredith Corp., 1716 Locust St., Des Moines, IA 50309; (515) 284-3000

New Low-fat Favorites
Ruth Spear
New York, NY: Little, Brown and Company, 1998, 306 p.
Little, Brown and Company, 3 Center Plaza, Boston, MA 02108; (617) 277-0730

Secrets of Fat-free Italian Cooking
Sandra Woodruff, R.D.
Garden City Park, NY: Avery Publishing Group, 1996, 230 p.
Avery Publishing Group, 120 Old Broadway, Garden City Park, NY 11040; (516) 741-2155

Simple Vegetarian Pleasures
Jeanne Lemlin
New York, NY: HarperCollins Publishers, 1998, 319 p.
HarperCollins Publishers, 10 E. 53rd St., New York, NY 10022; (212) 207-7000

Skinny Mexican Cooking
Sue Spitler
Chicago, IL: Surrey Books, 1996, 147 p.
Surrey Books, 230 East Ohio Street, Suite 120, Chicago, IL 60611;
(800) 326-4430

Skinny Pizzas: Over 100 Low-fat, Easy-to-Make, Delicious Recipes for America's Favorite Fun Food—From an Original Roman Pizza to Trendy California-style Dishes
Barbara Grunes
Chicago, IL: Surrey Books, 1996, 174 p.
Surrey Books, 230 East Ohio Street, Suite 120, Chicago, IL 60611;
(800) 326-4430

Skinny Spices: 50 Nifty Homemade Spice Blends That Can Make Any Diet Delicious
E. L. Klein
Chicago, IL: Surrey Books, 1990, 204 p.
Surrey Books, 230 East Ohio Street, Suite 120, Chicago, IL 60611;
(800) 326-4430

Food Composition Books (in alphabetical order by title)

Bowes & Church's Food Values of Portions Commonly Used, 17th edition, revised
Jean A. T. Pennington
Philadelphia, PA: Lippincott, Williams & Wilkins 1998, 481 p.
Lippincott, Williams & Wilkins, 227 E. Washington Sq., Philadelphia, PA 19106; (215) 238-4200

The Complete Book of Food Counts
Corinne T. Netzer
New York, NY: Dell Publishing, 1997, 770 p.
Dell Publishing, 1270 6th Ave., New York, NY 10020; (212) 698-1313

The Complete Food Count Guide
Editors of Consumer Guide, with the Nutrient Analysis Center, Chicago Center for Clinical Research
Lincolnwood, IL: Publications, Ltd., 1996, 704 p.
Publications, Ltd., 7373 N. Cicero Ave., Lincolnwood, IL 60646; (847) 676-3470

The Complete and Up-To-Date Fat Book. A Guide to the Fat Calories, and Fat Percentages in Your Food
Karen J. Bellerson
New York, NY: Avery Publishing Group, 1997, 870 p.
Avery Publishing Group, 120 Old Broadway, Garden City Park, NY 11040; (516) 741-2155

Fast Food Facts. The Original Guide for Fitting Fast Food into a Healthy Lifestyle
Marion J. Franz, MS, RD, LD, CDE
Minneapolis, MN: IDC Publishing, 1998, 243 p.
IDC Publishing, 3800 Park Nicollet Blvd., Minneapolis, MN 55416; (612) 993-3874

The Fat Counter. The Revised and Updated 4th edition
Annette B. Natow and Jo-Ann Heslin
New York, NY: Pocket Books, 1998, 661 p.
Pocket Books, 1230 Avenue of the Americas, New York, NY 10020; (212) 698-7000

Chapter 39

The Office of Research on Women's Health—ORWH

The following is an interview with Dr. Vivian Pinn, NIH Associate Director for Research on Women's Health. On November 19, 1991, Dr. Pinn was appointed Director of the newly formed Office of Research on Women's Health (ORWH). She discusses some of the major issues in women's health research and how ORWH is working to improve the health of American women.

Why was the Office of Research on Women's Health (ORWH) established at NIH and how does its mission fit into the research programs the institutes already have in place?

The office was established in the Office of the Director, NIH, in 1990, in response to a report by the U.S. General Accounting Office (GAO), mandated by the Congressional Caucus on Women's Issues, that women were routinely excluded from medical research supported by NIH. The report also stated that although NIH policy encouraged researchers to analyze study results by gender, the implementation of the policy for including women in research studies was not uniform or consistent. ORWH serves as the focal point for women's health research at NIH.

"Women's Health at NIH," from *News and Features*, Fall 1997, National Institutes of Health.

The office was charged with the task of carrying out three major mandates: to strengthen, develop, and increase research for women's health to eliminate gaps in knowledge, and determine the research agenda for women's health; to ensure that women are represented in NIH studies, especially clinical studies; and to increase the number of women in biomedical research careers. Although the Office of Research on Women's Health was charged with the primary responsibility for accomplishing these goals, this effort is a collaborative project with a shared responsibility with all the NIH institutes.

ORWH's task is to strengthen new initiatives, expand ongoing programs, and develop new ones, when appropriate. Shared funding allows ORWH to accomplish these goals by supporting research by co-funding projects and special initiatives through the various NIH components as well as co-sponsor scientific meetings to assist in determining the scientific agenda.

What are some of the knowledge gaps in women's health and how are they being addressed?

There is a need for basic information about normal, healthy development in girls and women across the lifespan as well as on diseases and conditions that primarily affect women, or those that affect both men and women but for which there is less research on women. We do know, for instance, that women tend to have more acute and chronic health problems than men. We also know that certain conditions are more prevalent in women than men, such as Alzheimer's disease, osteoporosis and certain immunologic disorders such as lupus. And although women tend to live longer than men they generally have more illnesses and disabilities than men. Perhaps insights into some of these fundamental questions will yield valuable information about the significance of sex/gender differences in health and disease that can improve our knowledge about the health of both men and women.

Traditionally, the concept of women's health focused on the reproductive system, especially during the childbearing years, without emphasizing the major non-reproductive diseases and illnesses that affect women. This narrow view of women's health was reflected in the underrepresentation of women in clinical studies of conditions that affect both men and women, but it also was an outgrowth of a biomedical research system that traditionally tended to view health and illness only in terms of the male model. We now know that research results obtained from studies on men do not always apply to women.

In recent years there has been an important shift in the traditional assumptions upon which the research model is based toward the inclusion of more women in research studies as well as a realization that gender differences need to be considered in the design and analysis of research studies. However, more needs to be done in this area. The NIH Office of Research on Women's Health, through a variety of mechanisms, has addressed these concerns by developing a comprehensive, broad-based research agenda for women's health that will expand basic, clinical, and applied research and ensure that women are appropriately represented in medical research studies.

How has the new, expanded definition of women's health made an impact on scientific research?

Because women's health research is no longer viewed solely in terms of reproductive health, the research agenda has broadened considerably to include areas that formerly were not always considered relevant to women's health. For example, we know that most women die of the same diseases as men: heart disease, cancer, and stroke, yet women were not always included in research studies on these diseases. Rather than think of diseases as specifically male or female, we've come to a realization that the same disease may have different manifestations that are gender specific and that these manifestations may provide important clues in the effort to improve disease diagnosis, treatment, and prevention. Moreover, research that includes women is producing new discoveries about the fundamental processes of health and disease in both men and women. For instance, we know that women are more vulnerable to autoimmune diseases than men, but we don't know why. Animal studies have shown the importance of hormonal and genetic factors in these disorders. A better understanding of autoimmunity in women can lead to a deeper understanding of the workings of the immune system in both genders.

Thus, in a very real sense, women's health research is changing the paradigm on which scientific research is based. Including women in research studies has generated a growing interest in gender-related research, which will lead to new opportunities to more accurately apply the results of research to greater numbers of people. This expanding field of research is not only attempting to identify gender differences and similarities with regard to health and disease, but also to determine the factors that lead to differences in health among different ethnic, racial, and other populations of women.

Finally, research strategies for women's health have begun to encompass a multidisciplinary perspective that reflects a growing awareness of the need to integrate women's health research into the framework of scientific research in order to benefit all Americans.

Why were women not included in research trials and what has NIH and ORWH done to ensure that they will be in the future?

There are no clear cut answers that fully explain why women were not included. It's also not clear that they were intentionally excluded, although certainly including women in research studies presented added complications, such as concerns that an experimental treatment or intervention would adversely affect an undetected pregnancy and that the menstrual cycle could confound results. We do know that women were not always included as participants in a number of large, landmark studies and that such exclusion is no longer considered acceptable without good reason.

> *"Ultimately, it is hoped that the results from research that includes women and minorities will move closer to closing the gap in scientific knowledge that currently exists with regard to these populations."*

It is interesting to note that guidelines for the inclusion of women have been in place at NIH since 1986. With the release of the GAO report the guidelines were revised and strengthened to ensure inclusion of women and minorities in NIH clinical studies. In 1993 they were revised again in response to the NIH Revitalization Act, thus making the NIH policy legally binding. The Act requires that women and minorities are included in clinical research and that clinical trials are designed and carried out to determine if the variables under study affect women and minorities differently from other subjects in the study. Exclusion is allowed if there is a substantial scientific rationale for doing so. Cost is not considered an acceptable justification for exclusion. In addition, outreach activities must be undertaken to recruit women and minorities as study participants.

These requirements were developed to allow investigators the opportunity to gather information on women and minorities early in the research process before interventions are developed so that gender and racial diversity can be taken into account in the final stages of research design and planning. Ultimately, it is hoped that the results from research that includes women and minorities will move closer to closing the gap in scientific knowledge that currently exists with regard to these populations.

How is NIH's Women's Health Initiative attempting to address the "knowledge gap" in women's health?

The Women's Health Initiative (WHI), which was announced in April, 1991, is one of the largest and most ambitious clinical studies ever conducted. The 15-year project will cost more than $635 million and is scheduled to involve more than 160,000 women ages 50-79, who will be studied at 40 clinical centers around the country. It has been characterized as "the most definitive, far-reaching study of women's health ever undertaken." The WHI will study ways to prevent the most common causes of death and disability among postmenopausal women: heart disease and stroke, cancer, and osteoporosis-related fractures. The WHI should redress some of the inequities that exist with regard to research as well as provide practical information for women and their physicians.

The study has two overall purposes. The first is to prevent cardiovascular disease, breast and colon cancer, and osteoporotic fractures, which are some of the major causes of death, disability, and frailty in older women. There are three components to this trial and women can enroll in more than one. One component will evaluate the effect of a low-fat diet in preventing heart disease and breast and colon cancer. Another will look at the effect of long-term hormone replacement therapy on heart disease and osteoporosis, and if there is any increased risk of breast cancer. A third arm of the study will evaluate the effect of calcium and vitamin D supplementation in preventing osteoporotic fractures and colon cancer.

Earlier, smaller studies found that some of these interventions may produce favorable results. Randomized, controlled, large scale trials, such as the WHI, provide conclusive data that can be translated to medical practice and to everyday life. Possible adverse effects from the interventions will be examined, as will the potential that some have additive effects, such as hormone replacement therapy and calcium supplementation on osteoporosis. Some women will not receive any specific interventions, but will be observed for an extended period of time to identify new risk factors that can predict the development of disease. The second part of the study, the community trial, will evaluate the effectiveness of various approaches in motivating older women to adopt healthy behaviors, such as healthy diets, smoking cessation, physical activity, and regular medical check-ups for early diagnosis of disease.

The WHI represents a major achievement in the effort to provide scientifically sound information for all women regardless of racial, cultural, or economic status. The information and benefits that will be obtained from the WHI studies will likely serve as the basis for disease prevention and health promotion programs that may significantly improve the health and well-being of future generations of women.

What are the implications of the genetic revolution for women's health and what opportunities lie ahead for scientific advancement of potential benefit to women?

The recent isolation of genes that predispose for breast and ovarian cancer provides great potential for increasing understanding of these diseases, and hopefully, for developing more effective prevention and treatments. For these and other diseases that affect women, the search for genes has opened up new areas of research on risk factors, heredity, and the relationship between genetics and the environment. When a disease gene is discovered, scientists have a powerful tool that can ultimately lead to novel and improved approaches to the prevention, detection, and treatment of disease based on more complete knowledge of underlying cellular and molecular mechanisms.

> *"The desire and the drive needed to pursue a career in scientific research has to be nurtured at an early age in the family and in schools where girls have their first exposures to science."*

The role of genetic factors, however, must be placed in proper perspective. The development of disease is a complex process and human beings are infinitely unique and varied in their response to their environment. Genetic information must be interpreted in light of individual differences. For instance, not all women with the genes that cause breast cancer—BRCA1 and BRCA2—will develop breast cancer. Those at greatest risk have a strong family history of the disease (a mother or sister with breast cancer). Further research is underway to determine the risk for women with a defective gene but without a family history. Since the majority of women who develop breast cancer do not have a defective gene, genetic susceptibility may be only one of several key factors in cancer development or undiscovered genes may be involved. Researchers continue to search for other genes involved in breast cancer and other cancers in women.

One issue that has raised considerable concern is the use of genetic testing for both high-risk and normal individuals. At meetings held in April and November, 1996, the Advisory Committee on Research on Women's Health of NIH's Office of Research on Women's Health discussed the issue of genetic testing for breast and ovarian cancer. In summary, the committee recommended that further research should be undertaken before genetic testing can be recommended for all women. High-risk women may receive more benefits from genetic testing, but more research is needed to determine if early medical interventions can reduce the risk of cancer in these women. The committee concluded that genetic testing should be provided in a research environment, which includes informed consent and counseling that addresses the current knowledge about genetic risk, available treatment options, and the limits of testing with respect to preventing disease.

The promise of genetic research is great, but it must be conducted with full knowledge and awareness of the social, ethical, and legal issues that affect the lives of the women who potentially benefit from this work. Research can never be conducted in a vacuum; it is a product of the society that supports it. We must proceed with the hope that genetic information will help us conquer disease by offering unparalleled opportunities to glimpse at and improve our future health. Public education, ethical standards, and societal involvement will help ensure that we use genetic information responsibly and wisely and for the benefit of all men and women.

An important mission of ORWH is to increase the representation of women in biomedical careers. How is NIH working toward this goal?

Unfortunately, women still face a number of obstacles that prevent them from entering and advancing in medical research careers. Women tend to select science careers less frequently than men do, and when they do so they often are paid less and experience more underemployment and unemployment than their male colleagues. Many of these problems are entrenched in a system that has been unwilling or unable to accommodate the needs of women with scientific careers. Much of this is due to the fact that society in general and the medical establishment in particular have not valued or encouraged young women to succeed in science nor has the dual role of women as family caregivers and professionals been appreciated. The desire and the drive needed to pursue a career in scientific research has to be nurtured at an early age in the family and in schools where girls have their first exposures to science. Reinforcement from mentors, colleagues, and institutions will offer significant benefits toward helping women stay "in the pipeline" rather than dropping out along the way.

The Office of Research on Women's Health believes that the best means of ensuring that research related to women's health remains a priority into the 21st century is to increase the number of women in leadership and policy-making positions in research and academic institutions both in the private and public sectors. Recruitment efforts have increased the numbers of women in medical and graduate schools, but comparable progress has not been made in the area of career advancement. In 1992, ORWH held a public hearing and workshop to determine the barriers and recommend solutions to increase the participation of women in scientific careers. As a result, ORWH developed and supported a number of initiatives to implement recommendations made at the workshop.

One important initiative—the ORWH Reentry Program—was developed in 1992 to assist fully trained scientists, the majority of whom are women, reestablish their careers in medical research after taking off time to attend to family responsibilities, such as caring for children. To date, more than 30 reentering scientists have participated in this program, which is supported by 17 NIH institutes. An evaluation of the program revealed that a majority of participants felt that the program had contributed to their long-term career goals. More extensive career follow-up of this and other programs will ensure that we are helping women overcome the barriers that prevent them from full participation and advancement in scientific careers.

What is the future of women's health in this country?

The future of women's health will be a reflection of the future of this country, and perhaps even the world. Women are the majority gender in this country. In many countries, including our own, women also are on the forefront of social and cultural reform. The role of women in our society has surpassed traditional gender stereotypes, just as women's health research now includes so much more than research on reproductive functions. Truly, we can be hopeful that this trend will continue, but we also must be mindful that true equity means including women of all races and cultures as full participants in medical and behavioral research both as researchers and research subjects.

As we enter the next millennium, and indeed the next phase of women's health in this country, we must direct our efforts to the empowerment of all women by increasing their knowledge and involvement in health care and health research. We must all work for the day when each woman, armed with solid health information based on research, can become her own health care advocate. In the pursuit of these goals, NIH will continue to lead the way in research on women's health so that American women and women the world over can look forward to a healthier and brighter future.

—Mary Sullivan, public affairs specialist,
Office of the Director, Office of Communications,
and editor, NIH News & Features Magazine.

Editorial Note

For more information about the Office of Research on Women's Health, visit http://www4.od.nih.gov/orwh.

Index

Index

Page numbers followed by 'n' indicate a footnote. Page numbers in *italics* indicate a table or illustration.

A

Abela, G. S. 23
ACE inhibitors 149, 281
ACS *see* American Cancer Society
Activase (alteplase) 25
adolescents, depression in women 78
adrenaline 73
African Americans
  angina 160
  heart disease risk factors 14, 28, 156–57
  high blood pressure 5, 48
age factor
  blood cholesterol testing 51
  blood pressure medication 59
  cardiovascular disease 156
  depression 134
  heart disease in women 4, 101
  heart disease risk factor 11–13, 14
  heart rate chart 42
  high blood pressure 48
  menopause 63–72
  myocardial infarction 162
  physical activity 104

alcohol abuse
  depression 77
  heart disease risk factor 16, 28
alcohol use
  breast cancer 213
  heart disease risk factor 57, 199
  high blood pressure 49, 97, 146
  moderate drinking, described 57
  triglycerides 62
Allen, J. K. 22
alteplase 25
American Cancer Society (ACS)
  dietary advice 213
  smoking cessation 120
American Dietetic Association, contact information 287
American Heart Association
  contact information 287
  women and heart disease 5
American Heart Association Cookbook, 5th edition (Winston) 289
American Institute of Nutrition, contact information 288
American Journal of Cardiac Imaging 24
American Journal of Cardiography 22
American Journal of Medicine 24
American Lung Association, smoking cessation 120

Health Reference Series
COMPLETE CATALOG

AIDS Sourcebook, 1st Edition

Basic Information about AIDS and HIV Infection, Featuring Historical and Statistical Data, Current Research, Prevention, and Other Special Topics of Interest for Persons Living with AIDS

Along with Source Listings for Further Assistance

Edited by Karen Bellenir and Peter D. Dresser. 831 pages. 1995. 0-7808-0031-1. $78.

"One strength of this book is its practical emphasis. The intended audience is the lay reader . . . useful as an educational tool for health care providers who work with AIDS patients. Recommended for public libraries as well as hospital or academic libraries that collect consumer materials."
—*Bulletin of the Medical Library Association, Jan '96*

"This is the most comprehensive volume of its kind on an important medical topic. Highly recommended for all libraries." —*Reference Book Review, '96*

"Very useful reference for all libraries."
—*Choice, Association of College and Research Libraries, Oct '95*

"There is a wealth of information here that can provide much educational assistance. It is a must book for all libraries and should be on the desk of each and every congressional leader. Highly recommended."
—*AIDS Book Review Journal, Aug '95*

"Recommended for most collections."
—*Library Journal, Jul '95*

AIDS Sourcebook, 2nd Edition

Basic Consumer Health Information about Acquired Immune Deficiency Syndrome (AIDS) and Human Immunodeficiency Virus (HIV) Infection, Featuring Updated Statistical Data, Reports on Recent Research and Prevention Initiatives, and Other Special Topics of Interest for Persons Living with AIDS, Including New Antiretroviral Treatment Options, Strategies for Combating Opportunistic Infections, Information about Clinical Trials, and More

Along with a Glossary of Important Terms and Resource Listings for Further Help and Information

Edited by Karen Bellenir. 751 pages. 1999. 0-7808-0225-X. $78.

"Recommended reference source."
—*Booklist, American Library Association, Dec '99*

"A solid text for college-level health libraries."
—*The Bookwatch, Aug '99*

Cited in *Reference Sources for Small and Medium-Sized Libraries, American Library Association, 1999*

Alcoholism Sourcebook

Basic Consumer Health Information about the Physical and Mental Consequences of Alcohol Abuse, Including Liver Disease, Pancreatitis, Wernicke-Korsakoff Syndrome (Alcoholic Dementia), Fetal Alcohol Syndrome, Heart Disease, Kidney Disorders, Gastrointestinal Problems, and Immune System Compromise and Featuring Facts about Addiction, Detoxification, Alcohol Withdrawal, Recovery, and the Maintenance of Sobriety

Along with a Glossary and Directories of Resources for Further Help and Information

Edited by Karen Bellenir. 650 pages. 2000. 0-7808-0325-6. $78.

SEE ALSO *Drug Abuse Sourcebook, Substance Abuse Sourcebook*

Allergies Sourcebook

Basic Information about Major Forms and Mechanisms of Common Allergic Reactions, Sensitivities, and Intolerances, Including Anaphylaxis, Asthma, Hives and Other Dermatologic Symptoms, Rhinitis, and Sinusitis

Along with Their Usual Triggers Like Animal Fur, Chemicals, Drugs, Dust, Foods, Insects, Latex, Pollen, and Poison Ivy, Oak, and Sumac; Plus Information on Prevention, Identification, and Treatment

Edited by Allan R. Cook. 611 pages. 1997. 0-7808-0036-2. $78.

Alternative Medicine Sourcebook

Basic Consumer Health Information about Alternatives to Conventional Medicine, Including Acupressure, Acupuncture, Aromatherapy, Ayurveda, Bioelectromagnetics, Environmental Medicine, Essence Therapy, Food and Nutrition Therapy, Herbal Therapy, Homeopathy, Imaging, Massage, Naturopathy, Reflexology, Relaxation and Meditation, Sound Therapy, Vitamin and Mineral Therapy, and Yoga, and More

Edited by Allan R. Cook. 737 pages. 1999. 0-7808-0200-4. $78.

Alzheimer's, Stroke & 29 Other Neurological Disorders Sourcebook, 1st Edition

Basic Information for the Layperson on 31 Diseases or Disorders Affecting the Brain and Nervous System, First Describing the Illness, Then Listing Symptoms, Diagnostic Methods, and Treatment Options, and Including Statistics on Incidences and Causes

Edited by Frank E. Bair. 579 pages. 1993. 1-55888-748-2. $78.

"Nontechnical reference book that provides reader-friendly information."
— *Family Caregiver Alliance Update, Winter '96*

"Should be included in any library's patient education section." — *American Reference Books Annual, 1994*

"Written in an approachable and accessible style. Recommended for patient education and consumer health collections in health science center and public libraries." — *Academic Library Book Review, Dec '93*

"It is very handy to have information on more than thirty neurological disorders under one cover, and there is no recent source like it." — *Reference Quarterly, Reference and User Services Association, Fall '93*

SEE ALSO Brain Disorders Sourcebook

Alzheimer's Disease Sourcebook, 2nd Edition

Basic Consumer Health Information about Alzheimer's Disease, Related Disorders, and Other Dementias, Including Multi-Infarct Dementia, AIDS-Related Dementia, Alcoholic Dementia, Huntington's Disease, Delirium, and Confusional States

Along with Reports Detailing Current Research Efforts in Prevention and Treatment, Long-Term Care Issues, and Listings of Sources for Additional Help and Information

Edited by Karen Bellenir. 524 pages. 1999. 0-7808-0223-3. $78.

"Recommended reference source."
— *Booklist, American Library Association, Oct '99*

Arthritis Sourcebook

Basic Consumer Health Information about Specific Forms of Arthritis and Related Disorders, Including Rheumatoid Arthritis, Osteoarthritis, Gout, Polymyalgia Rheumatica, Psoriatic Arthritis, Spondyloarthropathies, Juvenile Rheumatoid Arthritis, and Juvenile Ankylosing Spondylitis

Along with Information about Medical, Surgical, and Alternative Treatment Options, and Including Strategies for Coping with Pain, Fatigue, and Stress

Edited by Allan R. Cook. 550 pages. 1998. 0-7808-0201-2. $78.

"... accessible to the layperson."
— *Reference and Research Book News, Feb '99*

Asthma Sourcebook

Basic Consumer Health Information about Asthma, Including Symptoms, Traditional and Nontraditional Remedies, Treatment Advances, Quality-of-Life Aids, Medical Research Updates, and the Role of Allergies, Exercise, Age, the Environment, and Genetics in the Development of Asthma

Along with Statistical Data, a Glossary, and Directories of Support Groups and Other Resources for Further Information

Edited by Annemarie S. Muth. 650 pages. 2000. 0-7808-0381-7. $78.

Back & Neck Disorders Sourcebook

Basic Information about Disorders and Injuries of the Spinal Cord and Vertebrae, Including Facts on Chiropractic Treatment, Surgical Interventions, Paralysis, and Rehabilitation

Along with Advice for Preventing Back Trouble

Edited by Karen Bellenir. 548 pages. 1997. 0-7808-0202-0. $78.

"The strength of this work is its basic, easy-to-read format. Recommended."
— *Reference and User Services Quarterly, American Library Association, Winter '97*

Blood & Circulatory Disorders Sourcebook

Basic Information about Blood and Its Components, Anemias, Leukemias, Bleeding Disorders, and Circulatory Disorders, Including Aplastic Anemia, Thalassemia, Sickle-Cell Disease, Hemochromatosis, Hemophilia, Von Willebrand Disease, and Vascular Diseases

Along with a Special Section on Blood Transfusions and Blood Supply Safety, a Glossary, and Source Listings for Further Help and Information

Edited by Karen Bellenir and Linda M. Shin. 554 pages. 1998. 0-7808-0203-9. $78.

"Recommended reference source."
— *Booklist, American Library Association, Feb '99*

"An important reference sourcebook written in simple language for everyday, non-technical users. "
— *Reviewer's Bookwatch, Jan '99*

Brain Disorders Sourcebook

Basic Consumer Health Information about Strokes, Epilepsy, Amyotrophic Lateral Sclerosis (ALS/Lou Gehrig's Disease), Parkinson's Disease, Brain Tumors, Cerebral Palsy, Headache, Tourette Syndrome, and More

Along with Statistical Data, Treatment and Rehabilitation Options, Coping Strategies, Reports on Current Research Initiatives, a Glossary, and Resource Listings for Additional Help and Information

Edited by Karen Bellenir. 481 pages. 1999. 0-7808-0229-2. $78.

"Recommended reference source."
— *Booklist, American Library Association, Oct '99*

SEE ALSO Alzheimer's, Stroke & 29 Other Neurological Disorders Sourcebook, 1st Edition

Breast Cancer Sourcebook

Basic Consumer Health Information about Breast Cancer, Including Diagnostic Methods, Treatment Options, Alternative Therapies, Help and Self-Help Information, Related Health Concerns, Statistical and Demographic Data, and Facts for Men with Breast Cancer

Along with Reports on Current Research Initiatives, a Glossary of Related Medical Terms, and a Directory of Sources for Further Help and Information

Edited by Edward J. Prucha. 600 pages. 2000. 0-7808-0244-6. $78.

SEE ALSO *Cancer Sourcebook for Women, 1st and 2nd Editions, Women's Health Concerns Sourcebook*

Burns Sourcebook

Basic Consumer Health Information about Various Types of Burns and Scalds, Including Flame, Heat, Cold, Electrical, Chemical, and Sun Burns

Along with Information on Short-Term and Long-Term Treatments, Tissue Reconstruction, Plastic Surgery, Prevention Suggestions, and First Aid

Edited by Allan R. Cook. 604 pages. 1999. 0-7808-0204-7. $78.

"Recommended reference source."
—*Booklist, American Library Association, Dec '99*

SEE ALSO *Skin Disorders Sourcebook*

Cancer Sourcebook, 1st Edition

Basic Information on Cancer Types, Symptoms, Diagnostic Methods, and Treatments, Including Statistics on Cancer Occurrences Worldwide and the Risks Associated with Known Carcinogens and Activities

Edited by Frank E. Bair. 932 pages. 1990. 1-55888-888-8. $78.

Cited in *Reference Sources for Small and Medium-Sized Libraries, American Library Association, 1999*

"Written in nontechnical language. Useful for patients, their families, medical professionals, and librarians."
—*Guide to Reference Books, 1996*

"Designed with the non-medical professional in mind. Libraries and medical facilities interested in patient education should certainly consider adding the *Cancer Sourcebook* **to their holdings. This compact collection of reliable information . . . is an invaluable tool for helping patients and patients' families and friends to take the first steps in coping with the many difficulties of cancer."**
—*Medical Reference Services Quarterly, Winter '91*

"Specifically created for the nontechnical reader . . . an important resource for the general reader trying to understand the complexities of cancer."
—*American Reference Books Annual, 1991*

"This publication's nontechnical nature and very comprehensive format make it useful for both the general public and undergraduate students." —*Choice, Association of College and Research Libraries, Oct '90*

New Cancer Sourcebook, 2nd Edition

Basic Information about Major Forms and Stages of Cancer, Featuring Facts about Primary and Secondary Tumors of the Respiratory, Nervous, Lymphatic, Circulatory, Skeletal, and Gastrointestinal Systems, and Specific Organs; Statistical and Demographic Data; Treatment Options; and Strategies for Coping

Edited by Allan R. Cook. 1,313 pages. 1996. 0-7808-0041-9. $78.

"An excellent resource for patients with newly diagnosed cancer and their families. The dialogue is simple, direct, and comprehensive. Highly recommended for patients and families to aid in their understanding of cancer and its treatment." —*Booklist Health Sciences Supplement, American Library Association, Oct '97*

"The amount of factual and useful information is extensive. The writing is very clear, geared to general readers. Recommended for all levels." —*Choice, Association of College and Research Libraries, Jan '97*

Cancer Sourcebook, 3rd Edition

Basic Consumer Health Information about Major Forms and Stages of Cancer, Featuring Facts about Primary and Secondary Tumors of the Respiratory, Nervous, Lymphatic, Circulatory, Skeletal, and Gastrointestinal Systems, and Specific Organs

Along with Statistical and Demographic Data, Treatment Options, Strategies for Coping, a Glossary, and a Directory of Sources for Additional Help and Information

Edited by Edward J. Prucha. 1,100 pages. 2000. 0-7808-0227-6. $78.

Cancer Sourcebook for Women, 1st Edition

Basic Information about Specific Forms of Cancer That Affect Women, Featuring Facts about Breast Cancer, Cervical Cancer, Ovarian Cancer, Cancer of the Uterus and Uterine Sarcoma, Cancer of the Vagina, and Cancer of the Vulva; Statistical and Demographic Data; Treatments, Self-Help Management Suggestions, and Current Research Initiatives

Edited by Allan R. Cook and Peter D. Dresser. 524 pages. 1996. 0-7808-0076-1. $78.

". . . written in easily understandable, non-technical language. Recommended for public libraries or hospital and academic libraries that collect patient education or consumer health materials."
—*Medical Reference Services Quarterly, Spring '97*

"Would be of value in a consumer health library. . . . written with the health care consumer in mind. Medical jargon is at a minimum, and medical terms are explained in clear, understandable sentences."
—*Bulletin of the Medical Library Association, Oct '96*

325

"The availability under one cover of all these pertinent publications, grouped under cohesive headings, makes this certainly a most useful sourcebook."
— *Choice, Association of College and Research Libraries, Jun '96*

"Presents a comprehensive knowledge base for general readers. Men and women both benefit from the gold mine of information nestled between the two covers of this book. Recommended."
— *Academic Library Book Review, Summer '96*

"This timely book is highly recommended for consumer health and patient education collections in all libraries." — *Library Journal, Apr '96*

SEE ALSO Breast Cancer Sourcebook, Women's Health Concerns Sourcebook

Cancer Sourcebook for Women, 2nd Edition

Basic Consumer Health Information about Specific Forms of Cancer That Affect Women, Including Cervical Cancer, Ovarian Cancer, Endometrial Cancer, Uterine Sarcoma, Vaginal Cancer, Vulvar Cancer, and Gestational Trophoblastic Tumor; and Featuring Statistical Information, Facts about Tests and Treatments, a Glossary of Cancer Terms, and an Extensive List of Additional Resources

Edited by Edward J. Prucha. 600 pages. 2000. 0-7808-0226-8. $78.

SEE ALSO Breast Cancer Sourcebook, Women's Health Concerns Sourcebook

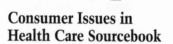

Cardiovascular Diseases & Disorders Sourcebook, 1st Edition

Basic Information about Cardiovascular Diseases and Disorders, Featuring Facts about the Cardiovascular System, Demographic and Statistical Data, Descriptions of Pharmacological and Surgical Interventions, Lifestyle Modifications, and a Special Section Focusing on Heart Disorders in Children

Edited by Karen Bellenir and Peter D. Dresser. 683 pages. 1995. 0-7808-0032-X. $78.

". . . comprehensive format provides an extensive overview on this subject."
— *Choice, Association of College and Research Libraries, Jun '96*

". . . an easily understood, complete, up-to-date resource. This well executed public health tool will make valuable information available to those that need it most, patients and their families. The typeface, sturdy non-reflective paper, and library binding add a feel of quality found wanting in other publications. Highly recommended for academic and general libraries. "
— *Academic Library Book Review, Summer '96*

SEE ALSO Healthy Heart Sourcebook for Women, Heart Diseases & Disorders Sourcebook, 2nd Edition

Communication Disorders Sourcebook

Basic Information about Deafness and Hearing Loss, Speech and Language Disorders, Voice Disorders, Balance and Vestibular Disorders, and Disorders of Smell, Taste, and Touch

Edited by Linda M. Ross. 533 pages. 1996. 0-7808-0077-X. $78.

"This is skillfully edited and is a welcome resource for the layperson. It should be found in every public and medical library." — *Booklist Health Sciences Supplement, American Library Association, Oct '97*

Congenital Disorders Sourcebook

Basic Information about Disorders Acquired during Gestation, Including Spina Bifida, Hydrocephalus, Cerebral Palsy, Heart Defects, Craniofacial Abnormalities, Fetal Alcohol Syndrome, and More

Along with Current Treatment Options and Statistical Data

Edited by Karen Bellenir. 607 pages. 1997. 0-7808-0205-5. $78.

"Recommended reference source."
— *Booklist, American Library Association, Oct '97*

SEE ALSO Pregnancy & Birth Sourcebook

Consumer Issues in Health Care Sourcebook

Basic Information about Health Care Fundamentals and Related Consumer Issues, Including Exams and Screening Tests, Physician Specialties, Choosing a Doctor, Using Prescription and Over-the-Counter Medications Safely, Avoiding Health Scams, Managing Common Health Risks in the Home, Care Options for Chronically or Terminally Ill Patients, and a List of Resources for Obtaining Help and Further Information

Edited by Karen Bellenir. 618 pages. 1998. 0-7808-0221-7. $78.

"The editor has researched the literature from government agencies and others, saving readers the time and effort of having to do the research themselves. Recommended for public libraries."
— *Reference and User Services Quarterly, American Library Association, Spring '99*

"Recommended reference source."
— *Booklist, American Library Association, Dec '98*

Contagious & Non-Contagious Infectious Diseases Sourcebook

Basic Information about Contagious Diseases like Measles, Polio, Hepatitis B, and Infectious Mononucleosis, and Non-Contagious Infectious Diseases like Tetanus and Toxic Shock Syndrome, and Diseases Occurring as Secondary Infections Such as Shingles and Reye Syndrome

Along with Vaccination, Prevention, and Treatment Information, and a Section Describing Emerging Infectious Disease Threats

Edited by Karen Bellenir and Peter D. Dresser. 566 pages. 1996. 0-7808-0075-3. $78.

Death & Dying Sourcebook

Basic Consumer Health Information for the Layperson about End-of-Life Care and Related Ethical and Legal Issues, Including Chief Causes of Death, Autopsies, Pain Management for the Terminally Ill, Life Support Systems, Insurance, Euthanasia, Assisted Suicide, Hospice Programs, Living Wills, Funeral Planning, Counseling, Mourning, Organ Donation, and Physician Training

Along with Statistical Data, a Glossary, and Listings of Sources for Further Help and Information

Edited by Annemarie S. Muth. 641 pages. 1999. 0-7808-0230-6. $78.

Diabetes Sourcebook, 1st Edition

Basic Information about Insulin-Dependent and Noninsulin-Dependent Diabetes Mellitus, Gestational Diabetes, and Diabetic Complications, Symptoms, Treatment, and Research Results, Including Statistics on Prevalence, Morbidity, and Mortality

Along with Source Listings for Further Help and Information

Edited by Karen Bellenir and Peter D. Dresser. 827 pages. 1994. 1-55888-751-2. $78.

". . . very informative and understandable for the layperson without being simplistic. It provides a comprehensive overview for laypersons who want a general understanding of the disease or who want to focus on various aspects of the disease."
— *Bulletin of the Medical Library Association, Jan '96*

Diabetes Sourcebook, 2nd Edition

*Basic Consumer Health Information about Type 1 Diabetes (Insulin-Dependent or Juvenile-Onset Diabetes), Type 2 (Noninsulin-Dependent or Adult-Onset Diabetes), Gestational Diabetes, and Related Disorders, Including Diabetes Prevalence Data, Management Issues, the Role of Diet and Exercise in Con-*trolling Diabetes, Insulin and Other Diabetes Medicines, and Complications of Diabetes Such as Eye Diseases, Periodontal Disease, Amputation, and End-Stage Renal Disease

Along with Reports on Current Research Initiatives, a Glossary, and Resource Listings for Further Help and Information

Edited by Karen Bellenir. 688 pages. 1998. 0-7808-0224-1. $78.

"Recommended reference source."
— *Booklist, American Library Association, Feb '99*

". . . provides reliable mainstream medical information . . . belongs on the shelves of any library with a consumer health collection."
— *E-Streams, Sep '99*

"Provides useful information for the general public."
— *Healthlines, University of Michigan Health Management Research Center, Sep/Oct '99*

Diet & Nutrition Sourcebook, 1st Edition

Basic Information about Nutrition, Including the Dietary Guidelines for Americans, the Food Guide Pyramid, and Their Applications in Daily Diet, Nutritional Advice for Specific Age Groups, Current Nutritional Issues and Controversies, the New Food Label and How to Use It to Promote Healthy Eating, and Recent Developments in Nutritional Research

Edited by Dan R. Harris. 662 pages. 1996. 0-7808-0084-2. $78.

"Useful reference as a food and nutrition sourcebook for the general consumer."
— *Booklist Health Sciences Supplement, American Library Association, Oct '97*

"Recommended for public libraries and medical libraries that receive general information requests on nutrition. It is readable and will appeal to those interested in learning more about healthy dietary practices."
— *Medical Reference Services Quarterly, Fall '97*

"An abundance of medical and social statistics is translated into readable information geared toward the general reader."
— *Bookwatch, Mar '97*

"With dozens of questionable diet books on the market, it is so refreshing to find a reliable and factual reference book. Recommended to aspiring professionals, librarians, and others seeking and giving reliable dietary advice. An excellent compilation."
— *Choice, Association of College and Research Libraries, Feb '97*

SEE ALSO *Digestive Diseases & Disorders Sourcebook, Gastrointestinal Diseases & Disorders Sourcebook*

Diet & Nutrition Sourcebook, 2nd Edition

Basic Consumer Health Information about Dietary Guidelines, Recommended Daily Intake Values, Vitamins, Minerals, Fiber, Fat, Weight Control, Dietary Supplements, and Food Additives

Along with Special Sections on Nutrition Needs throughout Life and Nutrition for People with Such Specific Medical Concerns as Allergies, High Blood Cholesterol, Hypertension, Diabetes, Celiac Disease, Seizure Disorders, Phenylketonuria (PKU), Cancer, and Eating Disorders, and Including Reports on Current Nutrition Research and Source Listings for Additional Help and Information

Edited by Karen Bellenir. 650 pages. 1999. 0-7808-0228-4. $78.

"Recommended reference source."
   —*Booklist, American Library Association, Dec '99*

SEE ALSO *Digestive Diseases & Disorders Sourcebook, Gastrointestinal Diseases & Disorders Sourcebook*

Digestive Diseases & Disorders Sourcebook

Basic Consumer Health Information about Diseases and Disorders that Impact the Upper and Lower Digestive System, Including Celiac Disease, Constipation, Crohn's Disease, Cyclic Vomiting Syndrome, Diarrhea, Diverticulosis and Diverticulitis, Gallstones, Heartburn, Hemorrhoids, Hernias, Indigestion (Dyspepsia), Irritable Bowel Syndrome, Lactose Intolerance, Ulcers, and More

Along with Information about Medications and Other Treatments, Tips for Maintaining a Healthy Digestive Tract, a Glossary, and Directory of Digestive Diseases Organizations

Edited by Karen Bellenir. 335 pages. 1999. 0-7808-0327-2. $48.

SEE ALSO *Diet & Nutrition Sourcebook, 1st and 2nd Editions, Gastrointestinal Diseases & Disorders Sourcebook*

Disabilities Sourcebook

Basic Consumer Health Information about Physical and Psychiatric Disabilities, Including Descriptions of Major Causes of Disability, Assistive and Adaptive Aids, Workplace Issues, and Accessibility Concerns

Along with Information about the Americans with Disabilities Act, a Glossary, and Resources for Additional Help and Information

Edited by Dawn D. Matthews. 600 pages. 2000. 0-7808-0389-2. $78.

Domestic Violence & Child Abuse Sourcebook

Basic Information about Spousal/ Partner, Child, and Elder Physical, Emotional, and Sexual Abuse, Teen Dating Violence, and Stalking, Including Information about Hotlines, Safe Houses, Safety Plans, and Other Resources for Support and Assistance, Community Initiatives, and Reports on Current Directions in Research and Treatment

Along with a Glossary, Sources for Further Reading, and Governmental and Non-Governmental Organizations Contact Information

Edited by Helene Henderson. 600 pages. 2000. 0-7808-0235-7. $78.

Drug Abuse Sourcebook

Basic Consumer Health Information about Illicit Substances of Abuse and the Diversion of Prescription Medications, Including Depressants, Hallucinogens, Inhalants, Marijuana, Narcotics, Stimulants, and Anabolic Steroids

Along with Facts about Related Health Risks, Treatment Issues, and Substance Abuse Prevention Programs, a Glossary of Terms, Statistical Data, and Directories of Hotline Services, Self-Help Groups, and Organizations Able to Provide Further Information

Edited by Karen Bellenir. 600 pages. 2000. 0-7808-0242-X. $78.

SEE ALSO *Alcoholism Sourcebook, Substance Abuse Sourcebook*

Ear, Nose & Throat Disorders Sourcebook

Basic Information about Disorders of the Ears, Nose, Sinus Cavities, Pharynx, and Larynx, Including Ear Infections, Tinnitus, Vestibular Disorders, Allergic and Non-Allergic Rhinitis, Sore Throats, Tonsillitis, and Cancers That Affect the Ears, Nose, Sinuses, and Throat

Along with Reports on Current Research Initiatives, a Glossary of Related Medical Terms, and a Directory of Sources for Further Help and Information

Edited by Karen Bellenir and Linda M. Shin. 576 pages. 1998. 0-7808-0206-3. $78.

"Overall, this sourcebook is helpful for the consumer seeking information on ENT issues. It is recommended for public libraries."
   —*American Reference Books Annual, 1999*

"Recommended reference source."
   —*Booklist, American Library Association, Dec '98*

Endocrine & Metabolic Disorders Sourcebook

Basic Information for the Layperson about Pancreatic and Insulin-Related Disorders Such as Pancreatitis, Diabetes, and Hypoglycemia; Adrenal Gland Disorders Such as Cushing's Syndrome, Addison's Disease, and Congenital Adrenal Hyperplasia; Pituitary Gland Disorders Such as Growth Hormone Deficiency, Acromegaly, and Pituitary Tumors; Thyroid Disorders Such as Hypothyroidism, Graves' Disease, Hashimoto's Disease, and Goiter; Hyperparathyroidism; and Other Diseases and Syndromes of Hormone Imbalance or Metabolic Dysfunction

Along with Reports on Current Research Initiatives

Edited by Linda M. Shin. 574 pages. 1998. 0-7808-0207-1. $78.

"Recommended reference source."
— *Booklist, American Library Association, Dec '98*

Environmentally Induced Disorders Sourcebook

Basic Information about Diseases and Syndromes Linked to Exposure to Pollutants and Other Substances in Outdoor and Indoor Environments Such as Lead, Asbestos, Formaldehyde, Mercury, Emissions, Noise, and More

Edited by Allan R. Cook. 620 pages. 1997. 0-7808-0083-4. $78.

"Recommended reference source."
— *Booklist, American Library Association, Sep '98*

"This book will be a useful addition to anyone's library." — *Choice Health Sciences Supplement, Association of College and Research Libraries, May '98*

". . . a good survey of numerous environmentally induced physical disorders . . . a useful addition to anyone's library."
— *Doody's Health Sciences Book Reviews, Jan '98*

". . . provide[s] introductory information from the best authorities around. Since this volume covers topics that potentially affect everyone, it will surely be one of the most frequently consulted volumes in the *Health Reference Series*." — *Rettig on Reference, Nov '97*

Ethical Issues in Medicine Sourcebook

Basic Information about Controversial Treatment Issues, Genetic Research, Reproductive Technologies, and End-of-Life Decisions, Including Topics Such as Cloning, Abortion, Fertility Management, Organ Transplantation, Health Care Rationing, Advance Directives, Living Wills, Physician-Assisted Suicide, Euthanasia, and More; Along with a Glossary and Resources for Additional Information

Edited by Helene Henderson. 600 pages. 2000. 0-7808-0237-3. $78.

Family Planning Sourcebook

Basic Information about Planning for Pregnancy and Contraception, Including Traditional Methods, Barrier Methods, Hormonal Methods, Permanent Methods, Future Methods, Emergency Contraception, Birth Control Choices for Women at Each Stage of Life, and Men's Role in Family Planning

Along with Statistics, Glossary, and Sources of Additional Information

Edited by Amy Marcaccio Keyzer. 600 pages. 2000. 0-7808-0379-5. $78.

SEE ALSO *Pregnancy & Birth Sourcebook*

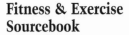

Fitness & Exercise Sourcebook

Basic Information on Fitness and Exercise, Including Fitness Activities for Specific Age Groups, Exercise for People with Specific Medical Conditions, How to Begin a Fitness Program in Running, Walking, Swimming, Cycling, and Other Athletic Activities, and Recent Research in Fitness and Exercise

Edited by Dan R. Harris. 663 pages. 1996. 0-7808-0186-5. $78.

"A good resource for general readers."
— *Choice, Association of College and Research Libraries, Nov '97*

"The perennial popularity of the topic . . . make this an appealing selection for public libraries."
— *Rettig on Reference, Jun/Jul '97*

Food & Animal Borne Diseases Sourcebook

Basic Information about Diseases That Can Be Spread to Humans through the Ingestion of Contaminated Food or Water or by Contact with Infected Animals and Insects, Such as Botulism, E. Coli, Hepatitis A, Trichinosis, Lyme Disease, and Rabies

Along with Information Regarding Prevention and Treatment Methods, and Including a Special Section for International Travelers Describing Diseases Such as Cholera, Malaria, Travelers' Diarrhea, and Yellow Fever, and Offering Recommendations for Avoiding Illness

Edited by Karen Bellenir and Peter D. Dresser. 535 pages. 1995. 0-7808-0033-8. $78.

"Targeting general readers and providing them with a single, comprehensive source of information on selected topics, this book continues, with the excellent caliber of its predecessors, to catalog topical information on health matters of general interest. Readable and thorough, this valuable resource is highly recommended for all libraries."
— *Academic Library Book Review, Summer '96*

"A comprehensive collection of authoritative information." — *Emergency Medical Services, Oct '95*

Food Safety Sourcebook

Basic Consumer Health Information about the Safe Handling of Meat, Poultry, Seafood, Eggs, Fruit Juices, and Other Food Items, and Facts about Pesticides, Drinking Water, Food Safety Overseas, and the Onset, Duration, and Symptoms of Foodborne Illnesses, Including Types of Pathogenic Bacteria, Parasitic Protozoa, Worms, Viruses, and Natural Toxins

Along with the Role of the Consumer, the Food Handler, and the Government in Food Safety; a Glossary, and Resources for Additional Help and Information

Edited by Dawn D. Matthews. 339 pages. 1999. 0-7808-0326-4. $48.

Forensic Medicine Sourcebook

Basic Consumer Information for the Layperson about Forensic Medicine, Including Crime Scene Investigation, Evidence Collection and Analysis, Expert Testimony, Computer-Aided Criminal Identification, Digital Imaging in the Courtroom, DNA Profiling, Accident Reconstruction, Autopsies, Ballistics, Drugs and Explosives Detection, Latent Fingerprints, Product Tampering, and Questioned Document Examination

Along with Statistical Data, a Glossary of Forensics Terminology, and Listings of Sources for Further Help and Information

Edited by Annemarie S. Muth. 574 pages. 1999. 0-7808-0232-2. $78.

"A wealth of information, useful statistics, references are up-to-date and extremely complete. This wonderful collection of data will help students who are interested in a career in any type of forensic field. It is a great resource for attorneys who need information about types of expert witnesses needed in a particular case. It also offers useful information for fiction and nonfiction writers whose work involves a crime. A fascinating compilation. All levels."
— *Choice, Association of College and Research Libraries, Jan 2000*

Gastrointestinal Diseases & Disorders Sourcebook

Basic Information about Gastroesophageal Reflux Disease (Heartburn), Ulcers, Diverticulosis, Irritable Bowel Syndrome, Crohn's Disease, Ulcerative Colitis, Diarrhea, Constipation, Lactose Intolerance, Hemorrhoids, Hepatitis, Cirrhosis, and Other Digestive Problems, Featuring Statistics, Descriptions of Symptoms, and Current Treatment Methods of Interest for Persons Living with Upper and Lower Gastrointestinal Maladies

Edited by Linda M. Ross. 413 pages. 1996. 0-7808-0078-8. $78.

"... very readable form. The successful editorial work that brought this material together into a useful and understandable reference makes accessible to all readers information that can help them more effectively under-

stand and obtain help for digestive tract problems."
— *Choice, Association of College and Research Libraries, Feb '97*

SEE ALSO *Diet & Nutrition Sourcebook, 1st and 2nd Editions, Digestive Diseases & Disorders Sourcebook*

Genetic Disorders Sourcebook

Basic Information about Heritable Diseases and Disorders Such as Down Syndrome, PKU, Hemophilia, Von Willebrand Disease, Gaucher Disease, Tay-Sachs Disease, and Sickle-Cell Disease, Along with Information about Genetic Screening, Gene Therapy, Home Care, and Including Source Listings for Further Help and Information on More Than 300 Disorders

Edited by Karen Bellenir. 642 pages. 1996. 0-7808-0034-6. $78.

"Recommended for undergraduate libraries or libraries that serve the public."
— *Science & Technology Libraries, Vol. 18, No. 1, '99*

"Provides essential medical information to both the general public and those diagnosed with a serious or fatal genetic disease or disorder."
— *Choice, Association of College and Research Libraries, Jan '97*

"Geared toward the lay public. It would be well placed in all public libraries and in those hospital and medical libraries in which access to genetic references is limited." — *Doody's Health Sciences Book Review, Oct '96*

Head Trauma Sourcebook

Basic Information for the Layperson about Open-Head and Closed-Head Injuries, Treatment Advances, Recovery, and Rehabilitation

Along with Reports on Current Research Initiatives

Edited by Karen Bellenir. 414 pages. 1997. 0-7808-0208-X. $78.

Health Insurance Sourcebook

Basic Information about Managed Care Organizations, Traditional Fee-for-Service Insurance, Insurance Portability and Pre-Existing Conditions Clauses, Medicare, Medicaid, Social Security, and Military Health Care

Along with Information about Insurance Fraud

Edited by Wendy Wilcox. 530 pages. 1997. 0-7808-0222-5. $78.

"Particularly useful because it brings much of this information together in one volume. This book will be a handy reference source in the health sciences library, hospital library, college and university library, and medium to large public library."
— *Medical Reference Services Quarterly, Fall '98*

Awarded "Books of the Year Award"
by the American Journal of Nursing, 1997

Health Resources Sourcebook

Basic Consumer Health Information about Sources of Medical Assistance, Featuring an Annotated Directory of Private and Public Consumer Health Organizations and Listings of Other Resources, Including Hospitals, Hospices, and State Medical Associations

Along with Guidelines for Locating and Evaluating Health Information

Edited by Dawn D. Matthews. 500 pages. 2000. 0-7808-0328-0. $78.

Healthy Aging Sourcebook

Basic Consumer Health Information about Maintaining Health through the Aging Process, Including Advice on Nutrition, Exercise, and Sleep, Help in Making Decisions about Midlife Issues and Retirement, and Guidance Concerning Practical and Informed Choices in Health Consumerism

Along with Data Concerning the Theories of Aging, Different Experiences in Aging by Minority Groups, and Facts about Aging Now and Aging in the Future; and Featuring a Glossary, a Guide to Consumer Help, Additional Suggested Reading, and Practical Resource Directory

Edited by Jenifer Swanson. 536 pages. 1999. 0-7808-0390-6. $78.

SEE ALSO Physical & Mental Issues in Aging Sourcebook

Healthy Heart Sourcebook for Women

Basic Consumer Health Information about Cardiac Issues Specific to Women, Including Facts about Major Risk Factors and Prevention, Treatment and Control Strategies, and Important Dietary Issues

Along with a Special Section Regarding the Pros and Cons of Hormone Replacement Therapy and Its Impact on Heart Health, and Additional Help, Including Recipes, a Glossary, and a Directory of Resources

Edited by Dawn D. Matthews. 400 pages. 2000. 0-7808-0329-9. $48.

SEE ALSO Cardiovascular Diseases & Disorders Sourcebook, 1st Edition, Heart Diseases & Disorders Sourcebook, 2nd Edition, Women's Health Concerns Sourcebook

Heart Diseases & Disorders Sourcebook, 2nd edition

Basic Consumer Health Information about Heart Attacks, Angina, Rhythm Disorders, Heart Failure, Valve Disease, Congenital Heart Disorders, and More, Including Descriptions of Surgical Procedures and Other Interventions, Medications, Cardiac Rehabilitation, Risk Identification, and Prevention Tips

Along with Statistical Data, Reports on Current Research Initiatives, a Glossary of Cardiovascular Terms, and Resource Directory

Edited by Karen Bellenir. 600 pages. 2000. 0-7808-0238-1. $78.

SEE ALSO Cardiovascular Diseases & Disorders Sourcebook, 1st Edition, Healthy Heart Sourcebook for Women

Immune System Disorders Sourcebook

Basic Information about Lupus, Multiple Sclerosis, Guillain-Barré Syndrome, Chronic Granulomatous Disease, and More

Along with Statistical and Demographic Data and Reports on Current Research Initiatives

Edited by Allan R. Cook. 608 pages. 1997. 0-7808-0209-8. $78.

Infant & Toddler Health Sourcebook

Basic Consumer Health Information about the Physical and Mental Development of Newborns, Infants, and Toddlers, Including Neonatal Concerns, Nutritional Recommendations, Immunization Schedules, Common Pediatric Disorders, Assessments and Milestones, Safety Tips, and Advice for Parents and Other Caregivers

Along with a Glossary of Terms and Resource Listings for Additional Help

Edited by Jenifer Swanson. 600 pages. 2000. 0-7808-0246-2. $78.

Kidney & Urinary Tract Diseases & Disorders Sourcebook

Basic Information about Kidney Stones, Urinary Incontinence, Bladder Disease, End Stage Renal Disease, Dialysis, and More

Along with Statistical and Demographic Data and Reports on Current Research Initiatives

Edited by Linda M. Ross. 602 pages. 1997. 0-7808-0079-6. $78.

Learning Disabilities Sourcebook

Basic Information about Disorders Such as Dyslexia, Visual and Auditory Processing Deficits, Attention Deficit/Hyperactivity Disorder, and Autism

Along with Statistical and Demographic Data, Reports on Current Research Initiatives, an Explanation of the Assessment Process, and a Special Section for Adults with Learning Disabilities

Edited by Linda M. Shin. 579 pages. 1998. 0-7808-0210-1. $78.

"Readable . . . provides a solid base of information regarding successful techniques used with individuals who have learning disabilities, as well as practical suggestions for educators and family members. Clear language, concise descriptions, and pertinent information for contacting multiple resources add to the strength of this book as a useful tool."
— Choice, Association of College and Research Libraries, Feb '99

"Recommended reference source."
— Booklist, American Library Association, Sep '98

"This is a useful resource for libraries and for those who don't have the time to identify and locate the individual publications."
— Disability Resources Monthly, Sep '98

■

Liver Disorders Sourcebook

Basic Consumer Health Information about the Liver and How It Works; Liver Diseases, Including Cancer, Cirrhosis, Hepatitis, and Toxic and Drug Related Diseases; Tips for Maintaining a Healthy Liver; Laboratory Tests, Radiology Tests, and Facts about Liver Transplantation

Along with a Section on Support Groups, a Glossary, and Resource Listings

Edited by Joyce Brennfleck Shannon. 591 pages. 2000. 0-7808-0383-3. $78.

■

Medical Tests Sourcebook

Basic Consumer Health Information about Medical Tests, Including Periodic Health Exams, General Screening Tests, Tests You Can Do at Home, Findings of the U.S. Preventive Services Task Force, X-ray and Radiology Tests, Electrical Tests, Tests of Blood and Other Body Fluids and Tissues, Scope Tests, Lung Tests, Genetic Tests, Pregnancy Tests, Newborn Screening Tests, Sexually Transmitted Disease Tests, and Computer Aided Diagnoses

Along with a Section on Paying for Medical Tests, a Glossary, and Resource Listings

Edited by Joyce Brennfleck Shannon. 691 pages. 1999. 0-7808-0243-8. $78.

"This is an overall excellent reference with a wealth of general knowledge that may aid those who are reluctant to get vital tests performed."
— Today's Librarian, Jan 2000

Men's Health Concerns Sourcebook

Basic Information about Health Issues That Affect Men, Featuring Facts about the Top Causes of Death in Men, Including Heart Disease, Stroke, Cancers, Prostate Disorders, Chronic Obstructive Pulmonary Disease, Pneumonia and Influenza, Human Immunodeficiency Virus and Acquired Immune Deficiency Syndrome, Diabetes Mellitus, Stress, Suicide, Accidents and Homicides; and Facts about Common Concerns for Men, Including Impotence, Contraception, Circumcision, Sleep Disorders, Snoring, Hair Loss, Diet, Nutrition, Exercise, Kidney and Urological Disorders, and Backaches

Edited by Allan R. Cook. 738 pages. 1998. 0-7808-0212-8. $78.

"Recommended reference source."
— Booklist, American Library Association, Dec '98

■

Mental Health Disorders Sourcebook, 1st Edition

Basic Information about Schizophrenia, Depression, Bipolar Disorder, Panic Disorder, Obsessive-Compulsive Disorder, Phobias and Other Anxiety Disorders, Paranoia and Other Personality Disorders, Eating Disorders, and Sleep Disorders

Along with Information about Treatment and Therapies

Edited by Karen Bellenir. 548 pages. 1995. 0-7808-0040-0. $78.

"This is an excellent new book . . . written in easy-to-understand language." *— Booklist Health Sciences Supplement, American Library Association, Oct '97*

". . . useful for public and academic libraries and consumer health collections."
— Medical Reference Services Quarterly, Spring '97

"The great strengths of the book are its readability and its inclusion of places to find more information. Especially recommended." *— Reference Quarterly, Reference and User Services Association, Winter '96*

". . . a good resource for a consumer health library."
— Bulletin of the Medical Library Association, Oct '96

"The information is data-based and couched in brief, concise language that avoids jargon. . . . a useful reference source." *— Readings, Sep '96*

"The text is well organized and adequately written for its target audience."
— Choice, Association of College and Research Libraries, Jun '96

". . . provides information on a wide range of mental disorders, presented in nontechnical language."
— Exceptional Child Education Resources, Spring '96

"Recommended for public and academic libraries."
— Reference Book Review, 1996

Mental Health Disorders Sourcebook, 2nd Edition

Basic Consumer Health Information about Anxiety Disorders, Depression and Other Mood Disorders, Eating Disorders, Personality Disorders, Schizophrenia, and More, Including Disease Descriptions, Treatment Options, and Reports on Current Research Initiatives

Along with Statistical Data, Tips for Maintaining Mental Health, a Glossary, and Directory of Sources for Additional Help and Information

Edited by Karen Bellenir. 605 pages. 2000. 0-7808-0240-3. $78.

■

Mental Retardation Sourcebook

Basic Consumer Health Information about Mental Retardation and Its Causes, Including Down Syndrome, Fetal Alcohol Syndrome, Fragile X Syndrome, Genetic Conditions, Injury, and Environmental Sources

Along with Preventive Strategies, Parenting Issues, Educational Implications, Health Care Needs, Employment and Economic Matters, Legal Issues, a Glossary, and a Resource Listing for Additional Help and Information

Edited by Joyce Brennfleck Shannon. 600 pages. 2000. 0-7808-0377-9. $78.

■

Obesity Sourcebook

Basic Consumer Health Information about Diseases and Other Problems Associated with Obesity, and Including Facts about Risk Factors, Prevention Issues, and Management Approaches

Along with Statistical and Demographic Data, Information about Special Populations, Research Updates, a Glossary, and Source Listings for Further Help and Information

Edited by Wilma Caldwell. 400 pages. 2000. 0-7808-0333-7. $48.

■

Ophthalmic Disorders Sourcebook

Basic Information about Glaucoma, Cataracts, Macular Degeneration, Strabismus, Refractive Disorders, and More

Along with Statistical and Demographic Data and Reports on Current Research Initiatives

Edited by Linda M. Ross. 631 pages. 1996. 0-7808-0081-8. $78.

■

Oral Health Sourcebook

Basic Information about Diseases and Conditions Affecting Oral Health, Including Cavities, Gum Disease, Dry Mouth, Oral Cancers, Fever Blisters, Canker Sores, Oral Thrush, Bad Breath, Temporomandibular Disorders, and other Craniofacial Syndromes

Along with Statistical Data on the Oral Health of Americans, Oral Hygiene, Emergency First Aid, Information on Treatment Procedures and Methods of Replacing Lost Teeth

Edited by Allan R. Cook. 558 pages. 1997. 0-7808-0082-6. $78.

"Unique source which will fill a gap in dental sources for patients and the lay public. A valuable reference tool even in a library with thousands of books on dentistry. Comprehensive, clear, inexpensive, and easy to read and use. It fills an enormous gap in the health care literature." — *Reference and User Services Quarterly, American Library Association, Summer '98*

"Recommended reference source."
— *Booklist, American Library Association, Dec '97*

Osteoporosis Sourcebook

Basic Consumer Health Information about Primary and Secondary Osteoporosis, Juvenile Osteoporosis, Related Conditions, and Other Such Bone Disorders as Fibrous Dysplasia, Myeloma, Osteogenesis Imperfecta, Osteopetrosis, and Paget's Disease

Along with Information about Risk Factors, Treatments, Traditional and Non-Traditional Pain Management, and Including a Glossary and Resource Directory

Edited by Allan R. Cook. 600 pages. 2000. 0-7808-0239-X. $78.

SEE ALSO *Women's Health Concerns Sourcebook*

■

Pain Sourcebook

Basic Information about Specific Forms of Acute and Chronic Pain, Including Headaches, Back Pain, Muscular Pain, Neuralgia, Surgical Pain, and Cancer Pain

Along with Pain Relief Options Such as Analgesics, Narcotics, Nerve Blocks, Transcutaneous Nerve Stimulation, and Alternative Forms of Pain Control, Including Biofeedback, Imaging, Behavior Modification, and Relaxation Techniques

Edited by Allan R. Cook. 667 pages. 1997. 0-7808-0213-6. $78.

"The text is readable, easily understood, and well indexed. This excellent volume belongs in all patient education libraries, consumer health sections of public libraries, and many personal collections."
— *American Reference Books Annual, 1999*

"A beneficial reference." — *Booklist Health Sciences Supplement, American Library Association, Oct '98*

"The information is basic in terms of scholarship and is appropriate for general readers. Written in journalistic style . . . intended for non-professionals. Quite thorough in its coverage of different pain conditions and summarizes the latest clinical information regarding pain treatment."
— *Choice, Association of College and Research Libraries, Jun '98*

"Recommended reference source."
— *Booklist, American Library Association, Mar '98*

Pediatric Cancer Sourcebook

Basic Consumer Health Information about Leukemias, Brain Tumors, Sarcomas, Lymphomas, and Other Cancers in Infants, Children, and Adolescents, Including Descriptions of Cancers, Treatments, and Coping Strategies

Along with Suggestions for Parents, Caregivers, and Concerned Relatives, a Glossary of Cancer Terms, and Resource Listings

Edited by Edward J. Prucha. 587 pages. 1999. 0-7808-0245-4. $78.

Physical & Mental Issues in Aging Sourcebook

Basic Consumer Health Information on Physical and Mental Disorders Associated with the Aging Process, Including Concerns about Cardiovascular Disease, Pulmonary Disease, Oral Health, Digestive Disorders, Musculoskeletal and Skin Disorders, Metabolic Changes, Sexual and Reproductive Issues, and Changes in Vision, Hearing, and Other Senses

Along with Data about Longevity and Causes of Death, Information on Acute and Chronic Pain, Descriptions of Mental Concerns, a Glossary of Terms, and Resource Listings for Additional Help

Edited by Jenifer Swanson. 660 pages. 1999. 0-7808-0233-0. $78.

"Recommended reference source."
—Booklist, American Library Association, Oct '99

SEE ALSO Healthy Aging Sourcebook

Plastic Surgery Sourcebook

Basic Consumer Health Information on Cosmetic and Reconstructive Plastic Surgery, Including Statistical Information about Different Surgical Procedures, Things to Consider Prior to Surgery, Plastic Surgery Techniques and Tools, Emotional and Psychological Considerations, and Procedure-Specific Information

Along with a Glossary of Terms and a Listing of Resources for Additional Help and Information

Edited by M. Lisa Weatherford. 400 pages. 2000. 0-7808-0214-4. $48.

Pregnancy & Birth Sourcebook

Basic Information about Planning for Pregnancy, Maternal Health, Fetal Growth and Development, Labor and Delivery, Postpartum and Perinatal Care, Pregnancy in Mothers with Special Concerns, and Disorders of Pregnancy, Including Genetic Counseling, Nutrition and Exercise, Obstetrical Tests, Pregnancy Discomfort, Multiple Births, Cesarean Sections, Medical Testing of Newborns, Breastfeeding, Gestational Diabetes, and Ectopic Pregnancy

Edited by Heather E. Aldred. 737 pages. 1997. 0-7808-0216-0. $78.

"A well-organized handbook. Recommended."
—Choice, Association of College and Research Libraries, Apr '98

"Reecommended reference source."
—Booklist, American Library Association, Mar '98

"Recommended for public libraries."
—American Reference Books Annual, 1998

SEE ALSO Congenital Disorders Sourcebook, Family Planning Sourcebook

---

Public Health Sourcebook

Basic Information about Government Health Agencies, Including National Health Statistics and Trends, Healthy People 2000 Program Goals and Objectives, the Centers for Disease Control and Prevention, the Food and Drug Administration, and the National Institutes of Health

Along with Full Contact Information for Each Agency

Edited by Wendy Wilcox. 698 pages. 1998. 0-7808-0220-9. $78.

"Recommended reference source."
—Booklist, American Library Association, Sep '98

"This consumer guide provides welcome assistance in navigating the maze of federal health agencies and their data on public health concerns."
—SciTech Book News, Sep '98

Rehabilitation Sourcebook

Basic Consumer Health Information about Rehabilitation for People Recovering from Heart Surgery, Spinal Cord Injury, Stroke, Orthopedic Impairments, Amputation, Pulmonary Impairments, Traumatic Injury, and More, Including Physical Therapy, Occupational Therapy, Speech/Language Therapy, Massage Therapy, Dance Therapy, Art Therapy, and Recreational Therapy

Along with Information on Assistive and Adaptive Devices, a Glossary, and Resources for Additional Help and Information

Edited by Dawn D. Matthews. 531 pages. 1999. 0-7808-0236-5. $78.

Respiratory Diseases & Disorders Sourcebook

Basic Information about Respiratory Diseases and Disorders, Including Asthma, Cystic Fibrosis, Pneumonia, the Common Cold, Influenza, and Others, Featuring Facts about the Respiratory System, Statistical and Demographic Data, Treatments, Self-Help Management Suggestions, and Current Research Initiatives

Edited by Allan R. Cook and Peter D. Dresser. 771 pages. 1995. 0-7808-0037-0. $78.

"Designed for the layperson and for patients and their families coping with respiratory illness. . . . an extensive array of information on diagnosis, treatment, management, and prevention of respiratory illnesses for the general reader." — *Choice, Association of College and Research Libraries, Jun '96*

"A highly recommended text for all collections. It is a comforting reminder of the power of knowledge that good books carry between their covers."
— *Academic Library Book Review, Spring '96*

"A comprehensive collection of authoritative information presented in a nontechnical, humanitarian style for patients, families, and caregivers."
— *Association of Operating Room Nurses, Sep/Oct '95*

Sexually Transmitted Diseases Sourcebook

Basic Information about Herpes, Chlamydia, Gonorrhea, Hepatitis, Nongonoccocal Urethritis, Pelvic Inflammatory Disease, Syphilis, AIDS, and More

Along with Current Data on Treatments and Preventions

Edited by Linda M. Ross. 550 pages. 1997. 0-7808-0217-9. $78.

Skin Disorders Sourcebook

Basic Information about Common Skin and Scalp Conditions Caused by Aging, Allergies, Immune Reactions, Sun Exposure, Infectious Organisms, Parasites, Cosmetics, and Skin Traumas, Including Abrasions, Cuts, and Pressure Sores

Along with Information on Prevention and Treatment

Edited by Allan R. Cook. 647 pages. 1997. 0-7808-0080-X. $78.

". . . comprehensive, easily read reference book."
— *Doody's Health Sciences Book Reviews, Oct '97*

SEE ALSO *Burns Sourcebook*

Sleep Disorders Sourcebook

Basic Consumer Health Information about Sleep and Its Disorders, Including Insomnia, Sleepwalking, Sleep Apnea, Restless Leg Syndrome, and Narcolepsy

Along with Data about Shiftwork and Its Effects, Information on the Societal Costs of Sleep Deprivation, Descriptions of Treatment Options, a Glossary of Terms, and Resource Listings for Additional Help

Edited by Jenifer Swanson. 439 pages. 1998. 0-7808-0234-9. $78.

"Recommended reference source."
— *Booklist, American Library Association, Feb '99*

"A useful resource that provides accurate, relevant, and accessible information on sleep to the general public. Health care providers who deal with sleep disorders patients may also find it helpful in being prepared to answer some of the questions patients ask."
— *Respiratory Care, Jul '99*

Sports Injuries Sourcebook

Basic Consumer Health Information about Common Sports Injuries, Prevention of Injury in Specific Sports, Tips for Training, and Rehabilitation from Injury

Along with Information about Special Concerns for Children, Young Girls in Athletic Training Programs, Senior Athletes, and Women Athletes, and a Directory of Resources for Further Help and Information

Edited by Heather E. Aldred. 624 pages. 1999. 0-7808-0218-7. $78.

Substance Abuse Sourcebook

Basic Health-Related Information about the Abuse of Legal and Illegal Substances Such as Alcohol, Tobacco, Prescription Drugs, Marijuana, Cocaine, and Heroin; and Including Facts about Substance Abuse Prevention Strategies, Intervention Methods, Treatment and Recovery Programs, and a Section Addressing the Special Problems Related to Substance Abuse during Pregnancy

Edited by Karen Bellenir. 573 pages. 1996. 0-7808-0038-9. $78.

"A valuable addition to any health reference section. Highly recommended."
— *The Book Report, Mar/Apr '97*

". . . a comprehensive collection of substance abuse information that's both highly readable and compact. Families and caregivers of substance abusers will find the information enlightening and helpful, while teachers, social workers and journalists should benefit from the concise format. Recommended."
— *Drug Abuse Update, Winter '96/'97*

SEE ALSO *Alcoholism Sourcebook, Drug Abuse Sourcebook*

Traveler's Health Sourcebook

Basic Consumer Health Information for Travelers, Including Physical and Medical Preparations, Transportation Health and Safety, Essential Information about Food, Water, Sun Exposure, Insect and Snake Bites, Camping and Wilderness Medicine, and Travel with Physical or Medical Disabilities

Along with International Travel Tips, Vaccination Recommendations, Geographical Health Issues, Disease Risks, a Glossary, and a Listing of Additional Resources

Edited by Joyce Brennfleck Shannon. 650 pages. 2000. 0-7808-0384-1. $78.

Women's Health Concerns Sourcebook

Basic Information about Health Issues That Affect Women, Featuring Facts about Menstruation and Other Gynecological Concerns, Including Endometriosis, Fibroids, Menopause, and Vaginitis; Reproductive Concerns, Including Birth Control, Infertility, and Abortion; and Facts about Additional Physical, Emotional, and Mental Health Concerns Prevalent among Women Such as Osteoporosis, Urinary Tract Disorders, Eating Disorders, and Depression

Along with Tips for Maintaining a Healthy Lifestyle

Edited by Heather E. Aldred. 567 pages. 1997. 0-7808-0219-5. $78.

"Handy compilation. There is an impressive range of diseases, devices, disorders, procedures, and other physical and emotional issues covered . . . well organized, illustrated, and indexed." —*Choice, Association of College and Research Libraries, Jan '98*

SEE ALSO *Breast Cancer Sourcebook, Cancer Sourcebook for Women, 1st and 2nd Editions, Healthy Heart Sourcebook for Women, Osteoporosis Sourcebook*

Workplace Health & Safety Sourcebook

Basic Information about Musculoskeletal Injuries, Cumulative Trauma Disorders, Occupational Carcinogens and Other Toxic Materials, Child Labor, Workplace Violence, Histoplasmosis, Transmission of HIV and Hepatitis-B Viruses, and Occupational Hazards Associated with Various Industries, Including Mining, Confined Spaces, Agriculture, Construction, Electrical Work, and the Medical Professions, with Information on Mortality and Other Statistical Data, Preventative Measures, Reproductive Risks, Reducing Stress for Shiftworkers, Noise Hazards, Industrial Back Belts, Reducing Contamination at Home, Preventing Allergic Reactions to Rubber Latex, and More

Along with Public and Private Programs and Initiatives, a Glossary, and Sources for Additional Help and Information

Edited by Chad Kimball. 600 pages. 2000. 0-7808-0231-4. $78.

■

Health Reference Series Cumulative Index, 1st Edition

A Comprehensive Index to the Health Reference Series, 1990-1999

1,500 pages. 2000. 0-7808-0382-5. $78.